THE *Non* RUNNER'S MARATHON GUIDE FOR WOMEN

GET OFF YOUR BUTT AND ON WITH YOUR TRAINING

Dawn Dais

SEAL PRESS

Published by Seal Press
A member of the Perseus Books Group
1700 4th Street
Berkeley, CA 94710

Library of Congress Cataloging-in-Publication Data

Dais, Dawn.
The nonrunner's marathon guide for women : get off your butt and on
with your training / Dawn Dais.
p. cm.
Includes bibliographical references and index.
ISBN-13: 978-1-58005-205-4 (alk. paper)
ISBN-10: 1-58005-205-3 (alk. paper)
1. Running for women. 2. Marathon running—Training. I. Title.

GV1061.18.W66N66 2006
796.42082—dc22

2006023886

20 19 18 17 16 15 14 13 12 11

Cover design by Gerilyn Attebery
Interior design by Megan Cooney
Printed in the United States of America by Berryville Graphics
Distributed by Publishers Group West

For my grandfather,
who never could have finished a marathon,
and who never would have doubted for one second that I could.

CONTENTS

Introduction

I bravely spent many months embedded in the marathon-training world. Much like the reporters who travel with soldiers during wartime, I barely made it out to tell my tale. What follows are my stories from the frontlines (or the backlines, as it were), as well as a training guide for those who want to follow in my recliner-to-race-day footsteps. How does one go from being a couch potato to finishing a marathon? One consumes a lot of ibuprofen.

Just like you may be starting your training, I began mine with my butt firmly attached to my recliner. After a little inspiration—and a lot of delusion—I hopped off that recliner and decided to run a marathon. Then reality set in (as it has a pesky way of doing), and I began to realize I was going to need a lot more than a little inspiration to get me through my months of training. Luckily, reality made an appearance about the same time my running buddy, Chipper Jen, did. I called her Chipper Jen because she was chipper as hell and had an enthusiasm for running that bordered on psychotic. Yet, her insane love of running and my insane running attempts somehow came together and helped us both through months of training and the marathon itself.

I'd like you to think of *The Nonrunner's Marathon Guide for Women* as your running buddy. It's here to keep you motivated and on the running trail when all you really want to do is lie on the couch and see what your TiVo has recorded for you. Rest assured that this book is much better than my running buddy; unlike Chipper Jen, this book will never call you at 6:30 AM on a friggin' Saturday and go on and on about how refreshing it is to run in the morning. This book is not a supporter of Saturday-morning chipperness.

Like any good running buddy though, it will relate to your running pain and will even bitch about it right along with you. As I began training, I also began keeping a journal of the highs (and quite a few lows). I've littered these journal entries throughout the book so that when you get tired of all the silly advice and information, you can just skip to one of my rants about muscle aches and/or spandex rashes and know that you're not alone in your training struggles.

While my journal entries tell my marathon story, the rest of *The Nonrunner's Marathon Guide for Women* is meant to help you begin to tell yours. (Hopefully your story won't involve as many curse words as mine.) I'm convinced that if I can finish a marathon, anyone else on the planet can, too. And I'm going to help you. I know it seems ridiculous. I know it seems impossible. I know that many cable services now offer video on demand, leaving you with no good reason to ever leave your love seat again. But I also know how great it can feel to get off your butt and challenge your body to do something other than set the world record for the least amount of calories burned in a day.

This book can help you attain marathon glory because it is unlike any other running book you will come across. Other books are written by elite runners who can run a marathon in the time it takes most of us to watch *The English Patient*. But *The Nonrunner's Marathon Guide for Women* is written by me, and I'm about as unelite as you're going to find. Why take marathon tips from a woman who is the self-proclaimed "worst runner in the world"? Because it's good for your self-esteem. When you're in Week 10 of your training and your feet suddenly turn into brick weights that you must drag along for miles at time, do you really think you'll find comfort and inspiration from a runner/author who could run from here to Argentina with a lethal combination of willpower and tremendous calf muscles? No, you need someone whose lack of real running talent or inclination will make you feel great about your own mediocre skills. And I am just that someone to make you feel like a star.

Your road to stardom begins with the training schedule (see pages 5–15) that was devised by my marathon coaches. The rest of the book offers advice on how to avoid death while training for a marathon. Keep in mind that my only real qualification for giving this advice is the fact that I managed to avoid death while training for a marathon. Which makes my training a smashing success. However, I issue this warning in case, for some odd reason, you actually follow my advice and something horrendous happens (like you end up actually enjoying running marathons): I hereby absolve myself from any liability.

So let's turn the page and get started on your road to the finish line. Get ready to test your limits, your drive, and your heart as you set out to accomplish a tremendous goal. In addition to this Oprah-esque stuff, you also might want to get ready to test your pain threshold, your PowerBar tolerance, and your comfort level with spandex on your butt. These are the things that will lead to the cursing I spoke of earlier. Good luck to you, soldier. . . .

Training Schedule

T*he Nonrunner's Marathon Guide for Women* provides you with lots of great advice from someone (that would be me) who has been in the trenches of marathon training and survived (barely) so that she could enlighten (or warn) others heading out to battle. But in addition to my wise advice and general sarcasm, readers may benefit from information from people who actually know what the hell they're talking about and don't gather most of their running facts while napping on park benches. That's where the coaches jog in.

Jeff Oberlatz and Michelle Mussuto are the two patient souls who coached me during my marathon. They are encyclopedias of running knowledge, as well as kick-ass runners in their own right. As they coached me, the most un-coachable person on the planet, they offered advice, but didn't push, and they were just all-around nice people. If I didn't associate them with knee pain, I'd probably have them over for dinner (and if I knew how to cook).

Following are marathon training schedules for walkers and run/walkers that Jeff and Michelle created. There's also a half-marathon training schedule if 13.1 miles seems plenty insane to you. Below the schedules you will find Jeff and Michelle's guidelines for how to decide whether you are a run/walker or a walker. Unfortunately, given my extensive athletic history, which only included throwing a shoe at the TV to change the channel because I lost the remote, I didn't fall into any category. So I just went with the run/walk method because I hear that variety is the spice of life. It is also the annihilator of muscles, as it turns out.

If you have the chance to train with real coaches, I hope you'll find some who are as patient and run-happy as Jeff and Michelle. And may I also suggest that you find some as good-looking as they, because during the times when you're lacking motivation and determination it's always helpful to have an attractive person to chase after. And you don't even have to worry about looking like a stalker. See, running can be fun.

Half-Marathon Training Schedule
RW=Run/Walker W=Walker

Week #	Sun	Mon	Tue	Wed	Thu	Fri	Sat
Week 1	You can, you will, you are able! And other motivational things!						
	RW: 35 min. W: 30 min.	Rest Day	RW: 35 min. W: 30 min.	RW: 40 min. W: 30 min.	Cross-Train 45 min.- 1 hour	Rest Day	RW: 45 min. W: 40 min.
Week 2	I'm getting a leg cramp just looking at this training schedule.						
	RW: 35 min. W: 30 min.	Rest Day	RW: 35 min. W: 30 min.	RW: 40 min. W: 30 min.	Cross-Train 45 min.- 1 hour	Rest Day	RW: 50 min. W: 45 min.
Week 3	Remember all that time you used to spend watching reruns on TV? That time is now spent moving. That is a bummer.						
	RW: 40 min. W: 35 min.	Rest Day	RW: 40 min. W: 35 min.	RW: 45 min. W: 40 min.	Cross-Train 45 min.- 1 hour	Rest Day	RW: 60 min. W: 50 min.

Week #	Sun	Mon	Tue	Wed	Thu	Fri	Sat
Week 4	Running seems like a fantabulous way to kill an hour on a Saturday.						
	RW: 50 min. / W: 40 min.	Rest Day	RW: 50 min. / W: 40 min.	RW: 55 min. / W: 45 min.	Cross-Train 45 min.-1 hour	Rest Day	RW: 60 min. / W: 60 min.
Week 5	If it hurts when you get out of bed in the morning, then you know you are training correctly.						
	RW: 40 min. / W: 40 min.	Rest Day	RW: 45 min. / W: 40 min.	RW: 40 min. / W: 35 min.	Cross-Train 45 min.-1 hour	Rest Day	RW: 90 min. / W: 75 min.
Week 6	Your body is probably pretty unhappy with you right now. It expresses its anger in the form of muscle aches and general immobility.						
	RW: 35 min. / W: 25 min.	Rest Day	RW: 45 min. / W: 35 min.	RW: 40 min. / W: 30 min.	Cross-Train 45 min.-1 hour	Rest Day	RW: 110 min. / W: 110 min.
Week 7	Are we having fun yet? Let me know if there is any fun planned, so I can be prepared.						
	RW: 45 min. / W: 45 min.	Rest Day	RW: 45 min. / W: 35 min.	RW: 40 min. / W: 35 min.	Cross-Train 45 min.-1 hour	Rest Day	RW: 3 miles / W: 3 miles
Week 8	Two months down. Many things on your body are probably feeling a little low as well.						
	RW: 4 miles / W: 3 miles	Rest Day	RW: 4 miles / W: 3 miles	RW: 5 miles / W: 4 miles	Cross-Train 45 min.-1 hour	Rest Day	RW: 5 miles / W: 4 miles

Week #	Sun	Mon	Tue	Wed	Thu	Fri	Sat
Week 9 Your recliner misses you.							
	RW: 4 miles **W:** 3 miles	Rest Day	**RW:** 5 miles **W:** 4 miles	**RW:** 5 miles **W:** 4 miles	Cross-Train 45 min.- 1 hour	Rest Day	6 miles
Week 10 Yes, Advil is a major food group.							
	4 miles	Rest Day	5 miles	3 miles	Cross-Train 45 min.- 1 hour	Rest Day	7 miles
Week 11 Are you eating a lot of carbs? 'Cause that's the only thing that makes any of this worth it.							
	4 miles	Rest Day	6 miles	3 miles	Cross-Train 45 min.- 1 hour	Rest Day	8 miles
Week 12 Wait, isn't training for a half-marathon supposed to be easier? This doesn't feel easy, does it?							
	5 miles	Rest Day	5 miles	3 miles	Cross-Train 45 min.- 1 hour	Rest Day	9 miles
Week 13 You can, you will, you are able (to eat a whole pizza and not gain weight).							
	4 miles	Rest Day	7 miles	5 miles	Cross-Train 45 min.- 1 hour	Rest Day	7 miles
Week 14 This is when a moped would start coming in handy.							
	4 miles	Rest Day	5 miles	3 miles	Cross-Train 45 min.- 1 hour	Rest Day	7 miles

Week #	Sun	Mon	Tue	Wed	Thu	Fri	Sat
Week 15	You can, you're able—oh crap, you have to run twelve miles next week!						
	5 miles	Rest Day	5 miles	4 miles	Cross-Train 45 min.-1 hour	Rest Day	7 miles
Week 16	Good news: You are only 1.1 miles away from the half-marathon. Bad news: You don't get credit for these twelve miles when you run your half-marathon.						
	3 miles	Rest Day	4 miles	4 miles	Cross-Train 45 min.-1 hour	Rest Day	12 miles
Week 17	You are on the homestretch now. Your body only has to stay upright for a few more weeks. Hang on.						
	4 miles	Rest Day	5 miles	5 miles	Cross-Train 45 min.-1 hour	Rest Day	6 miles
Week 18	*Aaaahhh*. Tapering is fun. By now your concept of fun is slightly askew.						
	5 miles	Rest Day	4 miles	5 miles	5 miles	Rest Day	4 miles
Week 19	Five days of rest in a row: The best five days of your training.						
	4 miles	4 miles	Rest Day	Rest Day	Rest Day	Rest Day	Rest Day
Week 20	This week is very important. If you don't follow the party schedule, then everything will fall apart.						
	RACE DAY	P	A	R	T	Y	!

Full Marathon Training Schedule
RW = Run/Walker   W = Walker

Week #	Sun	Mon	Tue	Wed	Thu	Fri	Sat
Week 1	You can, you will, you're able. And you look smashing in spandex.						
	RW: 35 min. / W: 30 min.	Rest Day	RW: 35 min. / W: 30 min.	RW: 40 min. / W: 30 min.	Cross-Train 45 min.-1 hour	Rest Day	RW: 45 min. / W: 40 min.
Week 2	You're hungry, you're tired, you're sore. And your spandex has given you an unfortunate rash.						
	RW: 35 min. / W: 30 min.	Rest Day	RW: 35 min. / W: 30 min.	RW: 40 min. / W: 30 min.	Cross-Train 45 min.-1 hour	Rest Day	RW: 50 min. / W: 45 min.
Week 3	Your body needs carbs and Advil, feed it lots, feed it often.						
	RW: 40 min. / W: 35 min.	Rest Day	RW: 40 min. / W: 35 min.	RW: 45 min. / W: 40 min.	Cross-Train 45 min.-1 hour	Rest Day	RW: 60 min. / W: 50 min.
Week 4	This is about the time your body starts realizing that this training stuff isn't just a phase. Be patient while it adjusts.						
	RW: 50 min. / W: 40 min.	Rest Day	RW: 50 min. / W: 40 min.	RW: 55 min. / W: 45 min.	Cross-Train 45 min.-1 hour	Rest Day	RW: 60 min. / W: 60 min.
Week 5	You are now moving for the running time of a movie. And you are equally as dramatic.						
	RW: 40 min. / W: 40 min.	Rest Day	RW: 45 min. / W: 40 min.	RW: 40 min. / W: 35 min.	Cross-Train 45 min.-1 hour	Rest Day	RW: 90 min. / W: 75 min.

Week #	Sun	Mon	Tue	Wed	Thu	Fri	Sat
Week 6	I bet those sore muscles are also starting to look a little toned. You are a running machine.						
	RW: 55 min. **W:** 45 min.	Rest Day	**RW:** 60 min. **W:** 50 min.	**RW:** 45 min. **W:** 40 min.	Cross-Train 45 min.-1 hour	Rest Day	**RW:** 115 min. **W:** 100 min.
Week 7	This is where we go from running times to running miles. This is when the fun starts to stop.						
	RW: 60 min. **W:** 50 min.	Rest Day	**RW:** 4 miles **W:** 3 miles	**RW:** 4 miles **W:** 3 miles	Cross-Train 45 min.-1 hour	Rest Day	**RW:** 6 miles **W:** 5 miles
Week 8	Two-month mark. Start valuing those rest days.						
	RW: 4 miles **W:** 3 miles	Rest Day	**RW:** 5 miles **W:** 4 miles	**RW:** 5 miles **W:** 4 miles	Cross-Train 45 min.-1 hour	Rest Day	**RW:** 7 miles **W:** 7 miles
Week 9	Double digits, baby! Most exclamation points this week will be after cuss words.						
	RW: 4 miles **W:** 3 miles	Rest Day	**RW:** 5 miles **W:** 5 miles	**RW:** 5 miles **W:** 4 miles	Cross-Train 45 min.-1 hour	Rest Day	10 miles
Week 10	Halfway home . . . if your home was, like, 300 miles away.						
	4 miles	Rest Day	4 miles	4 miles	Cross-Train 45 min.-1 hour	Rest Day	13 miles

Week #	Sun	Mon	Tue	Wed	Thu	Fri	Sat
Week 11	You will actually utter the words, "I only have to run nine miles this Saturday." My, how times have changed.						
	4 miles	Rest Day	4 miles	5 miles	Cross-Train 45 min.-1 hour	Rest Day	9 miles
Week 12	Do you think there is any possible way to gain without the pain? That would be awesome.						
	5 miles	Rest Day	3 miles	5 miles	Cross-Train 45 min.-1 hour	Rest Day	15 miles
Week 13	Seriously, didja ever think you'd say "Ran twenty miles," when someone asks, "What'd ya do this weekend?"						
	4 miles	Rest Day	3 miles	4 miles	Cross-Train 45 min.-1 hour	Rest Day	16 miles
Week 14	You are so close now, you can almost taste it. It tastes a lot like PowerBars.						
	4 miles	Rest Day	5 miles	4 miles	Cross-Train 45 min.-1 hour	Rest Day	18 miles
Week 15	Doesn't eight miles on Saturday seem quaint now?						
	4 miles	Rest Day	6 miles	5 miles	Cross-Train 45 min.-1 hour	Rest Day	8 miles
Week 16	Sweet Mary, some planes fly to destinations fewer miles away than this.						
	6 miles	Rest Day	5 miles	5 miles	Cross-Train 45 min.-1 hour	Rest Day	22 miles

Week #	Sun	Mon	Tue	Wed	Thu	Fri	Sat
Week 17 It's all about the tapering off. I excelled at the tapering.							
	4 miles	Rest Day	6 miles	5 miles	Cross-Train 45 min.- 1 hour	Rest Day	6 miles
Week 18 Your muscles are starting to get confused, "Why are you being so gentle?" Don't tell them, let them enjoy this time.							
	3 miles	Rest Day	3 miles	3 miles	Cross-Train 45 min.- 1 hour	Rest Day	5 miles
Week 19 Look at all the Rest Days. Best week ever.							
	5 miles	Rest Day	4 miles	Rest Day	Rest Day	Rest Day	Rest Day
Week 20 I have taken the liberty of filling in the rest of the week. If it's on the schedule, you have to do it.							
	RACE DAY	P	A	R	T	Y	!

WHERE DO I BEGIN?

Run/Walkers

- You should have some running (yes, jogging is okay) experience, which means you should have started running a few months ago.
- You should be able to run/walk at a conversational pace of twelve to fifteen minutes per mile.
- If you don't meet these criteria, you should definitely consider the walking schedule.

Walkers

- This schedule is for experienced walkers and coach potatoes alike.

- You should be able to walk at a fifteen-to-eighteen-minute-per-mile pace, what we like to call "walking with a purpose."
- If your pace is slower than nineteen minutes per mile, you should consider training for a marathon with a longer cut-off time.

Dawn's Note

There is no shame in training to walk. There is also no shame in training to run and being passed by the walkers (at least that's what I kept telling myself). I went with the run/walk method, even though I had no running experience. Of course, I lost both my kneecaps while training, and perhaps this was the reason why.

PICK THE EVENT THAT BEST FITS YOUR FITNESS LEVEL

Every marathon has a different cutoff time when the course closes and you'll be sharing the road with automobiles. The good news is that someone may offer you a ride. But if you're looking to actually cross the finish line on foot, make sure you pick an event that still has the finish line marked by the time you get to the end.

WHAT TRAINING IS REALLY ALL ABOUT

Consistency and low, incremental progress. Remember: The program is four to five months long to allow for adequate time to go from zero to 26.2, or 13.1!

- On shorter days, think of increasing your speed.

- During the week, you build endurance based on the frequency of your workouts, their intensity, and the time you spend working out.

- On weekends you build endurance based on increasing miles and time, and decreasing the intensity.

- Remember to take advantage of your rest days! It is important to rest to let the body heal and get you ready for the next day.

PAY ATTENTION TO YOUR FORM

Whether you run, run/walk, or walk, form is vital to staying healthy and helping to avoid injury.

- Keep your shoulders back.

- Keep your arms at ninety degrees—swing them like ski poles. Avoid crossing your chest.

- Open your chest (you want the maximum amount of oxygen available).

- Look toward the horizon.

- Keep your hands in lightly clenched fists.

Dawn's Note

Honestly, add in the spandex and the funny hat, and you've got no hope of looking cool while running. Keep looking at that horizon; don't pay any attention to the people laughing.

Now, enough with all this educated and professional advice, let's move on to the rest of the book!

THE
⋀PREPARATION

CHAPTER *One*
The Decision

Marathon training begins with making the actual decision to begin training. This involves differentiating between "I want to" and "I will." We all have lists, whether they be on paper or in our heads, of things we want to do: I want to visit all Seven Wonders of the World; I want to be a mom someday; I want to be bestest friends with Oprah Winfrey. Some wants are more attainable than others. I mean, if I asked Angelina Jolie, she'd probably tell me I can actually visit the Seven Wonders *and* get a kid at the same time. Of course, if I were to adopt a kid *with* Angelina Jolie, I might have a chance at the Oprah connection. . . .

The difference between "I want to" and "I will" lists usually lies in the amount of work inherently involved with the latter. Sometimes that work can quickly morph "I will" lists into "To hell with it" lists. Your job is to decide whether you're up to the work it takes to move marathon training to the "I will" list. This is not a decision to be taken lightly. This is the first "I will" in what will likely be a series of "I wills": I will go the entire day without being able to bend my leg; I will begin to dry heave at the mere mention of Gatorade; I will wonder if it is physically possible for my breasts to bounce off my body; and so on.

●●●

Ode to Running

What's the point of running?
What reason could there be?
Running twenty-six miles
Makes no sense to me.

We have planes, trains, and automobiles,
Helicopters, scooters, and boats.
And if you really, really need to
You could even ride a goat.

With all these options to move you
Why would you want to run?
Compared to running for hours
Riding a goat sounds like fun.

Running makes you sweaty
And tired and cranky and sore,
And running around in circles
Can be really quite a bore.

But the worst part of running,
What drives me out of my mind,
Are the Chipper Happy Runners
Who are Chipper and Happy all the time.

They get up at 7 AM
To run too many miles,
And whether it's Mile 1, 5, or 10,
Their faces are covered in smiles.

I fear that I'm outnumbered,
And they're trying to wear me down,
They're trying to make me chipper,
But all I can do is frown.

But I'll be nice to the Chipper People
And I'll tolerate their smiles,
'Cause they have so much friggin' energy
Maybe I can ride on their backs for a while.

To help in your decision-making process, I offer some easy-to-follow steps (none of which will answer the breast question—I leave that one up to you).

STEP 1: GET INFORMED

Marathon training isn't something to jump into on a whim. If you do, you're likely to crawl out of it on your hands and knees. Before you begin, be sure to get as much information as possible about what it entails. Well, actually, let me save you some time and give you my Cliff's Notes guide to marathon training: "Ouch," run ten miles; "I can't breathe," run fifteen miles; "My sports bra is slicing my body in half," collapse on a bag of ice at a race-day water station. The end.

Don't say I didn't warn you.

If you're considering training with a team, go to the informational session offered by the organization. Ask questions. Listen to the answers to other people's questions. Check to make sure the coach is cute. You know, get all the important information.

To really get an idea if you're ready to train for a marathon, take a look back at the training schedules (pages 6–13). Then look at them again. Don't just look at the 26.2-mile goal at the end of the training program. Look at the 300-plus miles you will have to run to *prepare* for the 26.2 miles. That's what'll getcha. The real miracle of training is not that you will have finished a marathon, but that you were even able to *start* the marathon after so many months of brutal training.

Now let's stop looking at the marathon schedule and start looking at some facts. The fact is that millions of people just like you have taken on the challenge of completing a marathon.

They have looked at a schedule similar to the one you've re-
viewed, and they too wondered how the hell they'd make it past
the third week without ending up on a stretcher. But somehow
they did it, and somehow you will, too. So as you are gathering
all of your information, and you are feeling completely and ut-
terly overwhelmed by it, remember that every marathoner felt
the same way at some point. If you're training with someone
who isn't overwhelmed, then they're most likely delusional and/
or extremely high. In either case, they probably aren't bad people
to know around Mile 20.

STEP 2: TAKE YOUR TIME

Before I began my journey to marathon glory, I had to decide
whether it was something I really wanted to do. This was a long
process for me. I was excited and pumped about the idea of
completing a marathon, but sometimes "excited and pumped"
can quickly be replaced by "hyperventilating and sore." And
that could happen during the very first mile of the very first
training run.

I have a checkered history of starting things and not finishing them (college, my great American novel, that broccoli on
my dinner plate). I grew tired of being the kind of person who
talked about doing things instead of actually doing them. I really
didn't want a marathon to be just one more of those things.

So when I got a postcard from the American Stroke
Association trying to lure me into marathon training, I thought
about it for a little while before I made my decision. I didn't
talk it over with anyone, didn't get other opinions. I simply sat
with the idea. I didn't want to utter the thought out loud until

I knew it was something I really wanted to do and not merely a momentary surge of enthusiasm.

I'm not saying you need to be as Secret Agent as I was. But I recommend letting the idea settle a bit before making your decision. As with any major choice, it's a good idea to sleep on it first. In fact, yes, do sleep on it. Because if you decide to train, that sleep is going to be your last ache-free slumber for a few months.

STEP 3: FIND A FRIEND

I'm sure there are some people who decide to train, read a how-to book, and a few months later cross the finish line. These people are not normal. Normal human beings are not equipped to endure chafing without the moral support of a fellow blistered being. It's just not in our nature.

As soon as you make your decision, I recommend finding a friend or group to train with. Numerous fundraising groups provide lots of support and guidance along the way, as well as the opportunity to raise money with your insane training. (See the Resources on page 243 for a listing of fundraising training groups.)

If raising money while trying to locate your missing knee-caps seems like too much to take on all at once, there are also many local running clubs that offer organized training and camaraderie that don't require you to hit up everyone you know for a great cause. I'm just as surprised as you that there are entire clubs devoted to running. In fact, there's a whole underground movement of runners you never knew existed—which is weird, because they mostly run above ground. Perhaps they run someplace other than the normal Taco Bell/Blockbuster/ home route I usually travel. A lot of local running stores have info on running groups, or you can go to the Road Runners Clubs of America website (www.rrca.org) for a listing of groups near you.

Big groups aren't the only way to train successfully. You can always form a group made up of friends. Just make sure they're as committed to the training as you are and will not be deterred by you calling to say, "I know we're supposed to run in like twenty minutes, but dammit if sushi doesn't sound better than a groin pull right now." The entire purpose of a running group is to keep you running. The only real requirement when picking a group is that members promise to convince you to get sushi *after* your run instead of *in place* of your run.

STEP 4: BE BOLD

After getting informed and taking your time and finding a friend or group to run with, it's now time to throw your hands up and say, "Screw it." Go ahead. Do it. Because if you're really going to train for a marathon, it inevitably means doing it against your better judgment. It's not going to make much sense; it's not going to seem possible that you signed yourself up to endure so much pain; and it's not going to be easy. Not even sorta. But one thing you'll learn after you cross the big finish line, and all the little finish lines in the middle, is that rarely will you find glory without struggle. The things that are easy? The things that make sense? Those aren't the things you talk about for years to come. They aren't the things you hang on your wall with pride. They *are* the things that will keep you from having to have knee-replacement surgery at age thirty, but we'll ignore that fact for the sake of inspiration right now.

When I was deciding whether to train, I had an overwhelming doubt that blanketed all my decision-making. All the "You can do it"s and the "Go girl"s were drowned out by "Uh, no you can't"s and the "Girl, you crazy"s running through my head. In the past, I'd experienced similar doubts and would back away from whatever was causing them. But when it came to the marathon, for the first time in my life I said, "Screw it," ignored the doubts, and went ahead with the training. (Interestingly, "Screw it" was the first in a long string of curse words that would exit my mouth during my training.)

Now that I've survived a marathon, I find myself purposely seeking out the things that bring me doubt, because I know that's where the glory lies. Can I promise that you won't fail in your marathon attempt? No. But I can promise that you won't succeed if you don't bother to try.

STEP 5: TELL EVERYONE YOU KNOW

Once you have defied logic and good sense and decided to train for a marathon, your next step is imperative: Tell every person you know (and even people you don't know) that you're training for a marathon. Not for the accolades or the sympathy or the awe. Do it for the accountability. Frankly, when you start to feel weak and sad and sore and broken, it's easier to just keep going than to try to explain why you quit. Quitting will make you feel bad enough. But reliving the shame every time someone asks, "How is the marathon thing going?" will truly suck. Believe me. The thought of telling friends and family I quit was enough to get me up from many a park bench.

Also, the accolades and the sympathy and the awe aren't bad either. One of the only consistently rewarding things about training is the consistently awed reactions you get from people when they hear about your endeavor. These people don't need to know you openly wept at Mile 14 last weekend, or that you can't bend over and pick up a pen off the floor. All they need to know is that you're awesome and deserve praise for your efforts. And all you need to know is that, yes, you are awesome. Screw the pen.

If you are still unsure about whether to train for a marathon, I've included a very helpful test that should clear up any lingering doubts:

THE "SHOULD I TRAIN FOR A MARATHON?" TEST

True or False

1. I have no real need to get anywhere when I run; I enjoy running for hours only to end up in the same place I started. **T / F**

2. Any sport in which people have been known to literally die of exhaustion while participating is just the kind of sport I've been looking for. **T / F**

3. I enjoy eating as many calories as I want and not gaining any weight. **T / F**

4. I'm interested in finding out exactly how many muscles I have in my legs. **T / F**

5. I have no problem being athletically inferior to someone twice my age. **T / F**

6. I've been sleeping in way too much, so I've been looking for something to take up a few hours on my Saturday mornings. **T / F**

7. I want to perfect the art of peeing in a shrub without being seen by anyone. **T / F**

8. My knee joints are overrated. **T / F**

9. I have no stairs in my home. **T / F**

10. Sometimes, when I'm driving long distances of, say, fifteen miles or so, I feel the overwhelming urge to pull my car over and simply run the rest of the way. **T / F**

11. I have a very good health plan. **T / F**

Multiple Choice

12. For a good time I prefer to
    a. Eat tacos.
    b. Watch TV.
    c. Watch TV while eating tacos.
    d. Run around in circles for four hours.

13. I prefer outfits that are
    a. Flattering.
    b. Inexpensive.
    c. Not full of holes.
    d. Skin-tight and rash-inducing.

14. One of my favorite things is
    a. Sleeping in on Saturday morning.
    b. Walking up a flight of stairs without taking a break in the middle.
    c. Having all my toenails intact.
    d. Training for a marathon.

If you answered "True" to Numbers 1–11 and "D" to Numbers 12–14, you are ready to train for a marathon! And to begin some sort of psychotherapy. So strap on those shoes, grab your water bottle, and jog down to your shrink's office! It's trainin' time!

If the test doesn't help you in your decision-making (and I can't imagine why it wouldn't) then I have another helpful tool: the good ol' pro/con list. This list will really help you organize your thoughts, get them down on paper, and weigh the pro side of the list against the con side. Try to be honest and to identify your personal pros and cons. I know the thought of that ibuprofen high and PowerBar diet will be overwhelmingly tempting. So be sure to balance them with some cons.

Here are some of my pros and cons:

PRO: I'll develop rock-solid abs.
CON: I'll need extra-strength ibuprofen.

PRO: I'll have a sense of accomplishment after I train.
CON: I'll have a sense of burning from all the chafing after I train.

PRO: I'll make new friends.
CON: I'll have limited time to spend with any friends because I'll be hospitalized with dehydration.

PRO: I'll be in the best shape of my life.
CON: I'll be in the most pain of my life.

PRO: I'll pay tribute to my grandfather.
CON: I'll have to pay someone to run the second half of the marathon for me.

PRO: I will challenge myself.
CON: I may hurt myself.

PRO: I'll raise money for a worthwhile cause.
CON: I may become a worthwhile cause after I fall into a
      sweat-induced coma.

PRO: I will get to shop for new clothes.
CON: I will be made to wear spandex.

PRO: I will gain respect (my own and other people's).
CON: I will gain blisters (in unfortunate and uncom-
      fortable places).

PRO: Seriously, did I mention the abs?

Below is space for you to complete your own pro/con list.
You might want to take yours a little more seriously than the one
I've outlined above because science has proven that sarcasm loses
its potency about 10.3 minutes into training. (That fact actually
turned out to be the biggest con on my list.) But all kidding aside,
the ab muscles are definitely a pro.

PRO: _____
_____

CON: _____
_____

PRO: _____
_____

CON: _____
_____

PRO: _____
_____

CON: _____
_____

Journal Entry: WEEK 1
Running 26.2 Miles—Best Idea Ever!

Wanna hear a joke? I'm gonna run a marathon. That's it. That's the punch line. It may not seem funny, but that's only because you haven't heard the setup. My name is Dawn, and prior to deciding to do this, I probably hadn't moved twenty miles in my life without the help of an automated device. A marathon is 26.2 miles. But we'll dwell on that insignificant detail later. More about my lifestyle first.

I work approximately six blocks from my house. It costs $50 a month to park in the office parking lot. A normal person with full use of her legs and senses would walk to work. I am not a normal person. My legs work fine, but my senses have never been in great shape. And those senses are disappointed every day at the end of my two-and-a-half-minute commute. Why? Because I park on the sixth floor and work on the seventh. Yes, mathematicians, that leaves one flight of stairs I have to walk up before I make it to work. It is almost more than I can take. I've thought about trying to get a parking permit for the lobby, which would eliminate the use of stairs altogether. I'm not sure how the receptionist would feel about me parking in front of her desk, but I'd be fine with it. I've never been a big fan of moving.

I'm a believer in the "don't run unless chased" philosophy of personal fitness. And even then, it really depends on who's doing the chasing. 'Cause let's be honest, I'm not going to outrun many people; so why not skip all that running and just get to the part where they catch me? A bit anticlimactic, yes, but much more energy efficient.

>>>

>>>

So, yeah, I'm gonna run a marathon. See, I told you it was funny.

How is it that I went from Elmer Fudd to the Road Runner? Well, I came home one day to find a postcard from the American Stroke Association in my mailbox. It showed very happy people very happily running a marathon to raise money for the American Stroke Association (hence their being featured on the association's postcard).

My grandfather had a debilitating stroke years ago and recently passed away. I sat staring at the postcard, feeling as if this were somehow a sign. "Do this marathon," he was saying. "Raise money for this cause."

There was also a coupon for Jimboy's Tacos in my mail. Apparently Grandpa was also saying, "Eat a discounted taco"—a message that seemed more his style.

But still, I could not ignore the sign. When you lose a relative, there's a feeling of wanting to do something—something huge and profound, something that honors a life that shaped and influenced your own. Though I knew I couldn't ever do anything big enough to honor his whole life, I figured this was something proactive and challenging and something that would have made my grandfather proud. And moving my lazy ass for twenty-six consecutive miles—that's pretty profound.

So that was that. I decided to run a marathon, or at least finish one. I would train hard and raise money and do something significant. Yes, that's what I would do!

When I shared this news with a few friends and family members their reactions were a mix of hysterical laughter, confusion, and then concern. Usually in that order. "Why would you do that?" "You can't do that."

>>>

>>>

"You hate running." "You still complain about the time I made you walk instead of drive to AMPM to get a Slurpee. And that was a block and a half." Others simply offered frowns and general perplexed looks.

My favorite reaction came from a woman who has known me for eighteen years. She looked at me and asked if I knew how much time, collectively, she had seen me run in the past eighteen years. "No," I replied. "About 3.2 seconds," she said flatly. "Dawn," she continued, "do you remember when we drove and drove and drove and drove to that restaurant I wanted to show you last month? That was about twenty-six miles." She looked triumphant. I've never really liked that woman, anyway.

Amazingly enough, these reactions made me even more resolute about my decision to train. Why? Because there is only one thing I can definitively say I am more than I am lazy, and that's stubborn. The best way to get me to do something is to tell me I can't.

So I attended the informational meeting about the marathon. I found out that there were two marathons in which I could run/crawl: one in Honolulu in December; the second in Arizona in January. Honolulu is a full marathon. Arizona gives runners the option of running either a full marathon or half-marathon and features one-hit wonder bands playing their songs at different points along the route. I'm thinking that basically everyone aims for the Honolulu Marathon, and the ones who can't quite cut it end up running the half-marathon in Arizona. And as they're running around the friggin' desert listening to "Unskinny Bop" for the tenth time, they're kicking themselves in the ass because they aren't running along a beach in Hawaii toward a pineapple drink and a cabana

>>>

>>>

boy awaiting them at the finish line. I'm aiming for the Honolulu Marathon. But I'm brushing up on my "Mambo No. 5" just in case.

Do I think I can really run a marathon? *Hmmm.* Physically, I know I can. Physically, I can do anything I set my mind to. It's the "set my mind to" part that might become a problem. But as I sat at the informational meeting and watched three people stand up when they asked if anyone training was a stroke survivor, I realized that there was no turning back. These people have trouble walking; some have partial paralysis of half their bodies. Some of them are here to train to walk a marathon. These people, like my grandfather once did, exert more effort getting dressed in the morning than I, an able-bodied person, do in an entire week. I owe it to them—and to my grandfather, and mostly to myself—to get off my ass and use this body I take for granted. And in doing so, I'll show my admiration and respect for those stroke survivors who are training alongside me, while raising money for stroke research. It seems like a win-win to me.

So this is where it all starts. The main goal is to not have a stroke while doing the marathon. It's important to dream big, you know.

CHAPTER *two*

The Reason

It is important to have at least one valid reason to do something insane—a reason that will hold up under scrutiny when sane people question your motives. But more important, the reason needs to hold up under your own scrutiny once the temporary effects of your spontaneity and/or pharmaceuticals wear off.

When deciding to train for a marathon, you actually need to have a very very good reason. Maybe even more than one very very good reason. Because that reason is going to be called upon repeatedly during the course of your training. At one point in your training, you'll find yourself lying on a park bench wanting to cry from the combination of pain, frustration, and exhaustion to which you've subjected your poor, defenseless body. But you know that crying will deplete your body of much-needed hydration and will probably cause your already-fatigued stomach muscles to tighten even more. As you lay there, a throbbing mess of pain and sweat, you will ask yourself how you got to this state and whether you'll ever again be able to function in a nonhorizontal fashion.

Self, you'll say (after rising at 6 AM to run for three hours, conversing with yourself will seem relatively sane), *why the hell are you doing this?* (Normally this phrase would end in an exclamation point, but you'll be too weak for an exclamation point.)

At this very moment you will need reasons, and they'll need to be rock-solid. Because anything even a little soft will be discarded as stupid and pointless and, "Oh my god, I must have been high to think that was a good reason." And that may lead to, "Oh my god, I wish I was high right now." And then the next thing you know, you've ditched this whole marathon idea and are following the latest incarnation of the Grateful Dead around the country.

So you see, it's important to have good reasons from the beginning—reasons that won't crack under pressure. One way to test them is to see how quickly you can come up with a relatively decent counterargument. Notice that the argument doesn't need to be great, just relatively decent. Because when you're lying on that bench, any argument will prove enough to talk you out of ever rising again.

Consider this example:

REASON:
I'm going to run this marathon to raise money for starving children.

EXHAUSTED-ON-A-BENCH COUNTERARGUMENT:
Well, the children are already starving. If I don't run this marathon, it's not like they are going to get any more hungry. But if I keep running today, I will definitely get hungrier. And that's not so much helping the problem as contributing to it. It's really my social responsibility to stop running right now.

Even starving children are not safe from the counterargument of an exhausted insane person.

To assist you in discovering your own reasons, I offer some I toyed with before finding reasons to get up from the bench and become a member of the vertical world once again:

REASON:
Running will help me get in shape.

EXHAUSTED-ON-A-BENCH COUNTERARGUMENT:
Who wants to be in shape? Why must I conform to society's idea of what my body should look like? I am woman, but I don't necessarily need to roar. I'm perfectly fine with the way I look. If god wanted me to look differently he wouldn't have invented recliners.

REASON:
I've always wanted to run a marathon.

EXHAUSTED-ON-A-BENCH COUNTERARGUMENT:
No I haven't.

REASON:
It will be great to set a goal and accomplish it, to feel a sense of pride when I cross a finish line.

EXHAUSTED-ON-A-BENCH COUNTERARGUMENT:
Since when do I set goals and actually accomplish them? And if I really feel the need to finish something, why don't I start with something a little less, I don't know, ridiculous? Why must I be so ambitious in my goal setting? Maybe I could set a goal to finish painting that garden gnome I started three years ago. The poor little guy is looking a bit pale.

REASON:
A bunch of my friends are training, too.

EXHAUSTED-ON-A-BENCH COUNTERARGUMENT:
I can get new friends.

REASON:
People will be really impressed if I finish a marathon.

EXHAUSTED-ON-A-BENCH COUNTERARGUMENT:
People would also be really impressed if I went on *Fear Factor* and won a hundred grand by eating cow

testicles. We obviously live in a society with low expectations. Maybe I could find a more stationary way to
impress people.

REASON:
No one thinks I can do it.

EXHAUSTED-ON-A-BENCH COUNTERARGUMENT:
Humph. Jerks. I'll show them. As soon as I can find my
kneecaps, I'll show them. In just a minute, I'll show them.
I just need one more minute and then they'd better look
out, 'cause I'm going to be showin'.

REASON:
I'm doing this as a fundraiser, and people have given me
money to do it.

EXHAUSTED-ON-A-BENCH COUNTERARGUMENT:
Well, it's not my fault people decided to sponsor a person
who can't even finish a damn garden gnome.

REASON:
This is a fundraiser for the American Stroke Association.
My late grandfather suffered a stroke years ago. I am do-
ing this in his memory.

EXHAUSTED-ON-A-BENCH COUNTERARGUMENT:
Ah, come on. Why did I have to pick this as a reason?
Who can let down a dead grandfather? Geez.

Throughout the weeks and months of training, I somehow
always found a reason to get up off the park bench. Sometimes
not until after I took a nap, but I eventually got up. Because I
knew the reasons (sometimes one of them, sometimes all of them)
to get up. I knew that I'm not a person who really cares about being in shape or what other people think, so those reasons weren't
going to work. And I knew that the promises I make to myself are

the easiest ones to break. ("Self, you were definitely high when you made that promise. Let's go grab some tacos and forget about this nonsense.")

But I also knew that if I made a promise to someone else, it would be nearly impossible for me to break it. In a small place inside me I made a promise to my grandfather to finish the race because he never could have. And, as I asked more and more people to sponsor my marathon, I was effectively promising I would actually *do* the marathon. So in the end, and in the middle, those people were the reasons I didn't quit.

I wish I could be more like Oprah and say that I did it for myself, that there was a hunger burning inside me to test my limits and roar right past them. But the only hunger came about twenty minutes after I stopped running, and the only burning came about twenty minutes after I wore a pair of spandex shorts that were a size too small.

On the following page, list your own reasons and exhausted-on-a-bench counterarguments. Make sure you come up with quite a few. Because as the weeks crawl by (or as you crawl by the weeks), you're going to need all the persuasion you can get. And don't forget to be honest with yourself. You know you aren't training for a marathon because you think you'll look smashing in running shorts. So don't put that down. Maybe you are training for a marathon because your coach *does* look smashing in running shorts. Go ahead and put that down.

● ● ●

REASON: _____

_____

EXHAUSTED-ON-A-BENCH COUNTERARGUMENT: _____

_____

_____

REASON: _____

_____

EXHAUSTED-ON-A-BENCH COUNTERARGUMENT: _____

_____

_____

REASON: _____

_____

EXHAUSTED-ON-A-BENCH COUNTERARGUMENT: _____

_____

_____

REASON: _____

_____

EXHAUSTED-ON-A-BENCH COUNTERARGUMENT: _____

_____

_____

REASON: _____

_____

EXHAUSTED-ON-A-BENCH COUNTERARGUMENT: _____

_____

_____

REASON: _____

_____

EXHAUSTED-ON-A-BENCH COUNTERARGUMENT: _____

_____

_____

Journal Entry: WEEK 5
Attacked!

I start Week 5 by running eleven miles—so compared to that, the rest of Week 5 is going smashingly. Yes, I just used the word "smashingly," even though I'm pretty sure only gay British men are allowed to use that word. But the point is, things can only get better when you start the week by running eleven miles. At 7 AM. On a Saturday. Wearing spandex. With Chipper Jen.

Actually, there have been a couple of disturbing incidents in Week 5. First, I was nearly attacked while running the other day. Well, maybe attacked isn't exactly the right word; but I think it's pretty accurate.

I was running along at my normal five-minute-mile pace (or maybe it was my five-minute-quarter-mile pace; whatever, it's not important) at a local park popular with runners and walkers alike. Apparently people like to run there because, oh, it's so cute, with the ducks and the roses and the adorable houses. That's what I have been told by Chipper Jen. I cannot confirm or deny the park's cuteness, because when I run I am aware of nothing at all, and I'm definitely not aware of anything adorable. A parade of puppies and newborns could go by and I wouldn't notice.

However, I do try to stay aware of the people around me. You know, in case someone is plotting to attack me. You never know when someone may jump out from behind the roses and hit me over the head with an adorable duck. It could happen.

So I'm running along and notice a man on a bike riding very slowly behind me. This seems weird because

>>>

>>>

(a) the man is well dressed, and (b) it is almost physically impossible to be going slower on a bike than I go as a runner. I was convinced that he was going to try to attack me. I was sure of it. I would definitely have to cut this run short. Of course, I was one of about thirty people jogging, so I guess the odds of him attacking me were slim. But he was wearing work clothes, so he was obviously not exercising on this trail populated with runners and walkers and adorable ducks. And you can never be too safe. So cutting my run short seemed to be the only safe thing to do.

Unfortunately, the well-dressed man passed me on his bike (i.e., he started pedaling). It appeared as though I was free from harm, but still, maybe I should cut the run short, as I was shaken from the near attack. No, I must be strong and continue on. Then I noticed another well-dressed man on a bike, riding very slowly. Clearly this attack was going to be a team effort.

The second man eventually passed me, too. Then, as I approached the end of one of my laps around the park, I saw that both of the men had stopped and were waiting on either side of the trail. Well, at least they were going to let me finish my mile. As I passed by the two men I could tell that they were trying to say something to me, but I didn't acknowledge them (i.e., I treated them like I do Chipper Jen). They were probably trying to tell me that they had planned to attack me. By ignoring them I had just barely escaped harm. I made another loop, and when I got to the end I could see that one of the well-dressed attackers was holding something in his hand, offering it to passing runners. Probably some sort of drug or weapon. As I got closer the man turned toward me, reached out his hand and ... offered me a Bible.

>>>

>>>

Turns out my attackers were Mormons trying to recruit at the local park. Apparently even god thinks I'm crazy. He is now sending his people to convince me of a better life than one spent running. I'll tell you one thing: I was on about Mile 4 when that guy offered me the Bible. Had he offered me his bike, I would have become a Mormon on the spot.

Terrifyingly, the Mormons weren't the only ones who posed a threat to me at the park. A few days later I made the mistake of joining the Stroke Association people for their weekly evening runs. Imagine fifteen Chipper Jens. Imagine them all coming at you at once. Imagine their catchphrases, their megaphones, their motivations, their encouragements. They were ten times scarier than the Mormons, in fact. The Mormons greeted me with a Bible. These people greeted me with, "So this is what we're gonna do. You are going to run your first mile at your pace; then when you run your second mile, you are going to try to cut ten seconds off your time; then on your third mile, try to cut fifteen seconds off your time." To this I replied, "How 'bout I run the first mile, then try not to get in my car and leave before I run the second mile, and then on the third mile I'll try not to pass out? These are more attainable goals for me."

Jen, of course, is in love with these people. These are *her* people. I guess if you like happy, friendly, warm, generous, and welcoming people, then you'd like them. I fear that I am now outnumbered when it comes to peppy people. They may try to lure me over to their side, just as the Mormons tried to lure me with a Bible. I will not be swayed. I will not let them bring me up to their level. Unless they offer me a bike.

CHAPTER *three*

The Accessories

Your accessory choices can really make or break your running experience. And I'm not saying that in a dramatic RuPaul sort of way. It's all fun and games until you have a bad sports bra that causes your boobs to chafe. Seriously, all good times end there.

The following is a list of all the accessories you'll need to be a successful runner. Well, you'll also need some running skill. And a high tolerance for muscle aches. And perhaps a personal masseuse. But this list should at least get you going in the right direction (that direction being that which does not lead you to chafed boobs).

SHOES

Shoes are probably the most important purchase you'll make. And the most expensive one as well. Resign yourself to the fact that you'll spend at least $100 on shoes. And more than likely you'll end up having to buy more than one pair before your training is over. I know, it sucks. Who knew running shoes can actually go bad? I didn't. Because I certainly never, ever had occasion to move enough to wear out anything—let alone a shoe.

Where to get them: Don't try to skimp, or your poor joints will end up paying for it. Go to your local running store and get to know one of its qualified Shoe People. I'm sure they have a title other than Shoe People, but that's what I call them, because they are the people who know all there is to know about shoes and feet and running and first-time runners who, without the aid of Shoe People, would wear Keds on seven-mile runs.

So have the Shoe People guide you to Your Perfect Pair of Shoes. Be prepared to have your foot poked and prodded and made to jog in the store. This is all in an attempt to prepare you for the impending humiliation you'll face when you step foot outside your house wearing spandex. Which leads us to . . .

RUNNING SHORTS

Running shorts come in various styles: You can get the baggy ones, the tight ones, the short ones (but please don't get short ones). Deciding which running shorts suit you best requires considering comfort and cosmetics. But it's difficult to find which shorts fit you well when you're trying them on in a dressing room. Like many running accessories, you won't really know if they're a good fit until you've run a couple miles in them. "Man, these things felt great in the dressing room, but now they have managed to rub off fourteen layers of the skin on my thigh."

I've tried all kinds of shorts and have found that I prefer the tight spandex-type shorts. They're not really visually appealing, but they're the only ones that don't cause me pain. And anything running-related that doesn't cause pain is always welcome.

I don't mind looser pants for shorter runs of only a couple of miles; but over the course of five to ten to fifteen miles, I get really tired of baggy shorts riding up and eventually forming a bulge of material in my crotch. Also, baggier shorts tend to rub more, causing a rash on the insides of my thighs that forces me to walk like a bull rider for a week. I know, I really have a way with visuals. It's a talent.

You might think that the short shorts eliminate the riding up, because they're already so short. And you'd be right. And at the same time, very, very wrong. Please understand that the sole purpose of running shorts is to cover your butt. That's why they are on this earth. So let's not deny them their purpose by making them so short that the butt can actually be seen peeking its way out. If you don't do it for the shorts, at least do it for your fellow runners.

Where to get them: You're gonna need quite a few pairs of running shorts; so I recommend buying them at a discount "dress for less" type store. You can also check out the discount rack while you are meeting with the Shoe People. I really don't see any reason to spend a lot of money on shorts. I mean, they're going to cover your butt whether you spend $40 or $10, right? (All nod in agreement because you're promising to never buy shorts that don't cover your butt.)

SPORTS BRAS

Sports bras are kinda like the boobs they hold—you don't really notice them until something goes wrong. In a perfect world, the first sports bra you purchase would be a perfect fit and become one with your body's movement. In the real world, it's hard to find the perfect sports bra; and even the perfect one takes awhile to become perfect. Like most of the clothes purchased for your running adventures, the sports bra is most likely going to get worse before it gets better.

Basically, running causes your body parts to move back and forth in a repetitive motion for hours at a time. This leads to a lot of rubbing, rubbing, and guess what, even more rubbing. Initially this causes pain, pain, and even more pain as your skin goes from being fresh and new to old and worn. But in between the new and old stages, it first gets red and causes you to gasp, "Oh my god, my body is just one open wound!" This is a completely natural part of the process, so don't freak out when you think you can see major organs peaking out from beneath your worn skin. This common runners' affliction is known as chafing.

Sports bras tend to cause the most chafing because they are usually the tightest thing you're wearing and have the most places to rub—under your armpits, under your boobs, on your shoulders, and even on your back. As much fun as sports bras are to wear, they're even more fun to take off. Houdini has nothing on a woman who can maneuver her way out of a sweat-soaked sports bra without breaking down in tears.

All this is to let you know you're not the only one who has battled (and lost to) a sports bra. Your goal should be to get all the battling out of the way before you hit the high mileage; 'cause when you're at Mile 18 and are battling fatigue, pain, dehydration, and the desire to call a cab, you do not want to be running with your arms straight out in an effort to avoid any more chafing in your armpits. My advice is to get a few sports bras and wear them in so that your body and your sports bra will be able to play well together when it counts.

If you have larger breasts, I recommend wearing two sports bras at one time. This may seem like overkill, but having boobs bouncing all over the place is not a good feeling or a good visual. I wore two the first month of training when all my body parts, including my breasts, were very unhappy about the bouncing taking place. Eventually my parts got used to it (also, there isn't nearly as much bouncing once you start to crawl), and I went back to wearing just one sports bra. But my ability to get out of *two* sports bras at a time still incites awe from all who hear the tale.

Where to get them: Sports bras can go either way. I've had really good ones that cost more than some people's car payments, and I've had good ones from a discount rack at a discount store. (Sure, they only had one armhole, but they were cheap!) It's hard to know what is going to fit your body best. Grab a variety of sports bras and take them for a spin. The one that draws the least amount of blood wins.

SOCKS

Who knew there were special kinds of socks for running? Who really cared? Well, you will after running a mile in bad socks. Your feet will be bloodied stumps where your beautiful soles once resided. And you will have to learn to navigate through the world by scooching on your behind, having lost use of the bottoms of your feet.

So scooch on down to the Shoe People and have them recommend socks. The Shoe People will warn you against cotton, which apparently will destroy your foot on contact. Or something like that. I've rarely seen anyone as passionate as my Shoe Person when he warned me about cotton socks. Apparently synthetic fibers are the way to go.

The next thing to look for in socks (seriously, did you ever think you'd have a list of things to look for in *socks?*) is whether they fit properly. You don't want them too loose or too tight. You want them juuuuust right. If you feel them bunching up around your feet (too loose) or can't feel your feet (too tight), then it's time to get a different pair of socks.

The socks I purchased had a double lining, which I was told would cause the sock to rub against itself instead of against my foot. I don't really understand how this works, but I'm sure my Shoe Person could give a detailed explanation. I had dinner plans that night so couldn't stick around for the sock lesson. I just took the socks and hoped they would rub against themselves instead of my feet. And they did. They were brilliant! That's why they cost $15, I'm guessing. But I never got a blister throughout my entire training. At least none on my feet . . .

Where to get them: Socks are important, so I recommend getting them where you get your shoes. Just pay your $15 and put it out of your mind as quickly as possible. Think of them as popcorn at a movie theater concession: They cost too much but in the end you are happier for having them.

SHIRTS

Shirts are another accessory that come in all shapes and sizes: loose ones, tight ones, short sleeved, long sleeved, no sleeved. Shirts are kind of a personal preference thing. And unlike short shorts, I have no strong feelings for or against running shirts, so I'll make no recommendation as to what type to purchase.

I will caution you to stay away from cotton and go for the synthetic fibers, which pull the sweat off your body (this is called wicking) and make it easier for your skin to breathe. Yeah, I have no idea how a shirt does that. I mean, it doesn't even plug into a wall or anything.

Where to get them: You'll need a lot of shirts so you might want to buy them at a discount store. Check the labels to make sure they aren't made out of cotton, and then be on your way. The half-off rack at the shoe store usually has some good shirts. And they have brand names, so they must be a lot better, right?

HATS

Hats are another item to pick up at the shoe store. Special running hats have holes all over the top and look quite aerodynamic. You have no idea how much heat your head puts off until you've run five miles wearing a hat with no holes. Holes create a little cooling system on top of your head (even though after you've run sixteen miles and sweated out every ounce of water in your body, your idea of "cool" is quite askew).

Where to get them: I've only seen these hats at running stores. As I don't think many nonrunners have much occasion to wear a hat with so many holes, it rivals a visor for effective top-of-the-head covering.

Journal Entry: WEEK 2
The Running Outfit

It's Week 2, and I'm happy to report I'm still alive. Although barely. I would like to start by clearing up a bit of confusion on the part of some of my more cynical friends and family members. The marathon to which I aspire is not a *Golden Girls* marathon on Lifetime or a *Real World* marathon on MTV or even a *Trading Places* marathon on TLC. It is an actual 26.2-mile running marathon on the island of Oahu. However, if someone would be willing to sponsor me for completing a TV-watching marathon, I might consider an event change.

But no, no, no, I'm running a marathon. Stop trying to distract me.

At the marathon information meeting I attended at the beginning of this whole thing, they gave me a mantra, "I can, I will, I am able." I was pumped up, I was inspired, I was motivated. Then I realized the marathon was going to involve some actual running. This deflated me just a little. How am I going to do this? How could I go from a near-comatose method of working out to running 26.2 miles? I realize that I have to start small—maybe with that pesky .2, then worry later about the other 26. Yes, that might work. If I gradually make my way up to 26.2 miles, maybe my body won't realize what is going on. And maybe I can occasionally hum *The Golden Girls* theme song so my body will think we're doing the kind of marathon it's used to.

But before any running could be done, I had to complete the most important part of the workout process:

>>>

>>>

the Running Outfit. Oh yes, people, one cannot properly exert energy without the proper attire. Plus, the day I spent shopping for the Running Outfit was one more day I could put off the Actual Running.

I made my way to the local running store, Fleet Feet, where a Fleet Footer helped me load up on all things marathonish. First, he pointed out the water bottle that straps around the waist. I was hoping for an IV hookup, but I guessed the strapping would have to do. Then there was the mesh hat, which is quite aerodynamic and will allow my head to "breathe" while running. Unfortunately, there was nothing for sale that would help the rest of my body breathe, but at least the top of my head wasn't going to hyperventilate. Next he showed me shirts and shorts, pointing out the ones made of synthetic fibers. "Cotton is rotten," he told me. Who knew? Then we got to the socks, synthetic as well. The pair he recommended had some special blah-blah, two layers of blah-blah that would help me with blah-blah. Whatever . . . I bought two pairs.

Lastly, we made our way to the shoe section. He asked me to jog briefly in the store so that he could determine the kind of shoes that would suit me best. I did the brief jog and tried my hardest to hide the fact that I was slightly winded from my ten-yard movement. He went in the back and emerged with several pairs of running shoes. I was disappointed to find that none of them had wheels on them. I was secretly hoping to slyly wheel past other marathoners just as kids wheel past me in the mall. With only wheel-less shoes to choose from, I made an educated, well-informed decision . . . and picked the ones that looked the best, of course.

>>>

> >>>
>
> So I was all set. I had all the hydrating, noncotton, aerodynamic items any marathoner could ever need. I made my way to the cash register where my total came to just under four grand. Well, I might be exaggerating a little, but not by much. But that's okay! You can't really put a price on the experience of completing a marathon. The experience of training and sweating and working and accomplishing. Well, Fleet Feet could put a price on it—and it does, and it's high. But that's okay! 'Cause "I can, I will, I am able" to pay for my Running Outfit.

WALKMAN/IPOD

A lot of times you'll be running with other people, and this is great. Because this means that they will provide you with conversation and stories and general distraction from what your body is going through. If you are running with other people and they are providing this distraction (some call it "camaraderie"), then you probably don't need a Walkman. And your friend who is going on and on about her date last night might actually be offended if you start listening to your collection of remixes during her story. But sometimes you are going to be running alone, and during those times you are going to need a Walkman or an iPod. Or you are going to go insane.

I'm tempted to put the Walkman and iPod at the very top of the accessory list because I think they're the single most important running accessory there is when you are running alone. You could technically run naked—no shoes or socks or shorts. But technically you cannot run without some sort of audio device when it's just you and the endless road ahead.

Because you will go nuts. (Which would probably be okay, considering you'd probably be sent to the crazy house for running naked.)

Get your iPod loaded with every song ever recorded or find a Walkman and get to know every channel on it. Whether it be rock, rap, country, or the public channel that's broadcast by two stoners with a microphone and an antenna. All these songs and stations will provide you with at least a little entertainment during your hours and hours of running.

The best-kept secret about Walkmans has got to be the AM channels. When the going gets tough, the tough surf the AM dial, where you'll find two beautiful things: sporting events and radio personalities who like the sound of their own voices. When you've been bouncing along for hours and your brain is completely void of new thoughts, AM radio can provide just enough mental stimulation to keep you from falling into a boredom-induced coma.

They say ("they" being the Organized Run Gods) that you can't wear a Walkman during organized runs. To that I say ("I" being the One Who Doesn't Follow Stupid Rules), "Hooey." Yes, *hooey*. Wear your Walkman, or study the entire *Encyclopaedia Britannica* before the race so that you'll have plenty of thoughts to keep you busy. Here's one thought you'll have: *Why the hell is* everyone *else wearing headphones and I'm not? Hooey.*

Where to get them: You can get an iPod at any electronics store, or you can probably use the one you have already. I should warn you that running is dirty and sweaty and wet and gross. And anything associated with running can become all those things. If you're going to take your beloved iPod out on the running trail, be extra careful not to get the grossness on it.

You can get a Walkman at any electronics store and some running stores. They're not very expensive and are remarkably durable. (For the sake of scientific experimentation, I dropped mine fifty-seven times and poured water on it thirteen times. Sure it got stuck on the same channel from time to time, but there was still sound coming out of the headphones, which was all I needed.) A lot of running stores sell Walkmans that fit on your bicep and make you look cool. I bought mine at the grocery store, because I was already wearing spandex and a hat with holes. Cool had passed me by weeks earlier, and I didn't expect it would be visiting ever again.

WATER-HOLDER BUTT THINGY

I'm sure it has a more technical name, but I call it the Water-Holder Butt Thingy. And essentially that's what it is: sort of a fanny pack that holds a water bottle. You clip it around your waist and have easy access to water at all times. This is quite helpful when you can see the water fountain on the horizon, but can't imagine having enough energy to get to it. Also, water fountains seem to get farther and farther apart as the run goes on; so it's nice to have a consistent water source, even during trying times.

Some people do not like the Water-Holder Butt Thingy. They think it bounces too much on their butt or doesn't hold enough water or makes their ass look too big. As I mentioned, I wear spandex, so I had to deal with the appearance of my ass long before I got to the water bottle. But if you want something different, there are other water-holding options: high-tech water bottles that don't even require you to tip them when drinking; backpack-style water bags with a little hose that fits over your shoulder to drink from. Hell, you could probably even put a beer hat on and drink water from it if you're so inspired (and so able to balance it). Water is a very important part of your effort to stay alive while training, so you need to find the least-annoying water-transporter for you and stick with it.

Where to get it: This is another running store item. It can also be found at sporting goods stores, because sporty people of all genres enjoy hydration. With a name like Water-Holder Butt Thingy, it's sure to gain popularity and start showing up in even more stores throughout the land.

WATCH

I was told to get a watch when I began training, so I'll tell you to get one too. To do variations of the run/walk method of training, you need to time your running and walking. Also, if you want to know how slowly or fast you're going, you'll need a watch to confirm your prowess. Truth be told, I lost my watch after the first week and didn't find it until a month after I finished the marathon. So I'm thinking it wasn't vital to my training or . . . its absence is what caused me to be the slowest runner ever. I'm sure that was it.

Where to get it: Any place that sells watches. I don't recommend spending an exorbitant amount on a watch that can calculate your cholesterol level in Japan, unless you're into that kind of

thing. In that case, you'll be giddy about the insanely complicated watches out there that can do everything short of your
laundry (which I find disappointing). If you're a techie, this
could be your time to shine. Some watches have GPS devices,
heart rate monitors, compasses, barometers that provide weather forecasts, timers that can save ninety-nine running times. The
list goes on and on. I could never find one that had wheels and
had no need for anything else, so a watch wasn't a high priority
for me.

GATORADE

I don't really know if you need Gatorade, but you need a sports
drink. And as a product of our commercially driven society, I
needed Gatorade. I filled my Water-Holder Butt Thingy with
Gatorade, then relied on water fountains for any water I wanted
during my run. I found a Gatorade flavor I liked and stuck with
it to the bitter end. At which point I promptly threw every
last ounce of the Gatorade mix away, vowing to never drink it
again. (If I can't be as athletic as the people on Gatorade commercials, I can at least be as dramatic.)

Where to get it: I bought Gatorade at a bulk store—one of
those places where everything is sold in packages of eighty-
two and you can eat a four-course meal while wandering the
aisles on Sample Day. I bought a huge tub of Gatorade mix
and mixed it before every run. This worked, until I put a bag
of powdered mix in my suitcase and it exploded over all my
clothes. But I hardly think it's fair to blame powdered sub-
stances for my stupidity.

GU

Vitamin-enriched GU Energy Gel is a goo-like substance that comes in little pouches. You rip one open, squirt it in your mouth, and you are hit with all sorts of energy and spirit. Or something. You aren't going to need GU right away; but you'll need it as the mileage gets longer and you start needing to replenish yourself. Some people call this point "Your body telling you to stop running." Runners call it "Time for GU."

Where to get it: I got mine at the running store, and can't imagine another place selling such a horrible, horrible invention. I mean, it's goo for god's sake. You can get it at some natural foods stores that cater to runner types, but I'm not thinking it's a huge seller in the supermarket chains.

BODYGLIDE

BODYGLIDE Skin Formula looks like deodorant and applies like deodorant, but it's not deodorant. You can tell, 'cause you never see people putting deodorant along their panty line and in their butt cracks. Not that there's anything wrong with that.

The basic purpose of BODYGLIDE is to, uh, help your body glide and prevent chafing. It rolls on like Vaseline and helps ease the discomfort of body parts and clothing rubbing together. Some people swear by it and lather themselves in it even if they're only walking to the car. Other people (yours truly) forget about it altogether until marathon day, then cover themselves with it from head to 'toe. Unfortunately, those people (yours truly) are morons, because while BODYGLIDE can make your body *parts* glide together a little easier, it does nothing to help with the overall gliding of your body. At Mile 15, the word "tumble" would probably be a better word to use than "glide" to describe what my body was doing.

Where to get it: You can buy it at the running store. Or if you want to go old school you can pick up some Vaseline and use that instead. But it doesn't come in a cute little roll-on package, so it probably doesn't work as well. Sometimes you can find a BODYGLIDE-type substance on big slabs of cardboard along the actual marathon course. People (Serious Runners) dip their hands into it and lather themselves as they run. I can't think of any possible way my body would ever be moving so vigorously as to require such on-the-move lathering.

Journal Entry: **WEEK 3**
It Takes More Than Just
the Running Outfit

Today I spent time lying on the floor having a heart to heart with my body. It seems that my muscles were under the impression that this current running craze was going to last as long as my other attempts at regular movement—about two weeks. They seemed to be humoring me the past couple of weeks, assuming they'd be back to lazy mode shortly. Upon realizing that this movement thing was becoming a regular occurrence, all of my muscles became very flustered and tightened up simultaneously in an attempt to voice their unanimous disapproval of the direction I was heading. We have yet to reach an acceptable compromise.

>>>

>>>

The running itself is going well, or as well as running can go. I basically run around in circles for minutes and sometimes hours at a time. No matter how far I run, it seems I always end up right back where I started from—circle after circle of running. If I ran in a straight line, I'd at least be somewhere near San Francisco by now with all the friggin' running I've done. But no, I just end up back at my car every single time. I keep myself motivated because I have a purpose: I am doing something greater than me—"I can, I will, I am able." Or something. I'm too busy trying not to pass out to remember catchphrases.

While I'm running, I notice there are other people out there too. I doubt all of them are being sponsored. So what the hell motivates them to run around in circles for minutes and hours at a time? I cannot even begin to fathom such motivation. These people annoy me. They're all, "Look at me. I can run past you twice in one lap." And, "I'm so special because I can carry on a conversation and run at the same time." And my favorite, "I'm the happiest damn runner you've ever seen. I never stop smiling. I just love, love, love running." I would hurt these people if I could catch them.

I found the sport to be rather boring, so I invested in some headphones to complete my Running Outfit. Although I can't change the fact that I'm basically running in the same circle for hours, I can change the radio station. One lap I run to a little 50 Cent, then Tim McGraw, followed by some Creedence Clearwater Revival. And it's always nice to know that Whitney will always love me. Listening to the radio, I inevitably have to listen to some DJs and commercials, because sometimes I just don't have the energy to change the station.

>>>

>>>

I have found these DJs and commercials to be quite informative, though. For instance, did you know that there are more than four hundred laxatives on the market? Now you do. Did you know that a man carried a refrigerator a hundred miles on a dare? Or that some yoga classes let people bring their dogs? Or that Carrie from Elk Grove wants to send a shout out to her supersweet boyfriend, Ryan? Didja know? Didja care? Probably not. I've learned one thing that definitely needs to be shared: Nighttime radio hosts on soft rock stations need to be shot. There is a local DJ who hosts 8 PM Love Songs on weeknights. Now I'm not saying this guy is boring. He very well might have plenty of interesting things to say. But, it takes him forty-five minutes to utter each syllable. The man has been trying to form a sentence since 1982.

Another addition to my running routine is my friend Chipper Jen. She's not just a Happy Runner, she's overall a pretty happy person. I love her to death; she's a great person, a great friend, with a great heart. But I may have to kill her. She is all, "You can do it. It's mind over matter. Just one more mile. It's so beautiful out here. Good job. I'll run backward in front of you to encourage you along."

Again, if I had the energy, I'd hurt her. I did, however, muster up the energy to tell her that people training for marathons often lose their toenails. This turned Chipper Jen into Toenail-Paranoid Chipper Jen—still chipper, but absolutely terrified of losing her toenails. This turned me into Amused Dawn.

Another big change in my routine: I have been eating better and drinking lots of water. Or at least I'm trying to. I've been a bit hot and cold when it comes to the newfound healthy diet. On the one hand, I have

>>>

>>>

a refrigerator full of healthy whatnots, which I've been eating for breakfast, lunch, and dinner. On the other hand, I took my eight-year-old cousin Katy to the state fair the other day and proceeded to eat all things deep-fried, including a deep-fried SNICKERS bar. Why deep-fry a SNICKERS bar? you might ask. Why not? I may answer. I'm a strong supporter of deep-frying pretty much anything edible and some things inedible. And being a woman of conviction, I'm not about to let some pesky marathon training get in the way of the things I stand for. That conviction would also explain the somewhat unhealthy diet I maintained on a recent camping trip. And by "somewhat" I mean "completely."

Yet I don't think my weekend off the healthy wagon was all lost. Just as I am challenging myself to run a marathon I also challenged myself to survive only on Tostitos and Tostitos Cheese Dip for three days. Through a lot of hard work and determination, I was able to do it. It was especially trying toward the end of the weekend when I was down to the chip crumbs and the bottom of the jar of cheese. I had to maneuver the crumbs in such a way as to scrape the remaining cheese without getting my hand stuck in the cheese jar. Fortunately, I have quite a few years of training for that event and was able to come away unscathed.

Following the weekend of chips and cheese, I decided I should probably invest in some vitamins. Although I'm sure Tostitos makes a vitamin-packed product, I thought maybe a multivitamin might supply those one or two important nutrients that tortilla chips lack. I was told to go to Costco to buy them because, like my Running Outfit, vitamins don't come cheap. But unlike my Running Outfit, vitamins are in an aisle

>>>

>>>

just past the bulk candy aisle. Whose idea was this?! After I loaded a forty-five-pack of sour straws into my cart, I made my way to the healthy aisle.

Chipper Jen had told me to look for a multivitamin and a vitamin by the name of "glucosamine," which is supposed to help my knees and other joints. Instead of glucosamine, I've always used the popular "sit-on-my-ass-amine" vitamin, and my knees have never hurt. But whatever. I'm a new visitor to the healthy aisle, who am I to judge?

I found glucosamine, which advertises on its label, "For Healthy Joints*." The multivitamin I chose pictures good-looking, happy, healthy people on the label and promises that "This product contains a scientifically designed blend of vitamins, minerals, and herbs that work together to help your body maintain healthy energy levels, endure the effects of life's stress, promote overall well-being.*" Notice the asterisks on both labels? They both relate to this disclaimer: "*These statements have not been evaluated by the Food and Drug Administration." So basically instead of saying "For Healthy Joints*" the glucosamine label could just as easily read "Strap one of these to your ass and you will fly to the moon.*" As long as they have the handy little asterisk, they can write whatever they want on the front of their bottle. They might as well write, "We don't really know what these pills do, but we know that idiots like you will spend a small fortune buying them as long as we put pictures of good-looking people with rock-hard abs on the bottle. Take two daily.*" I bought both bottles.

JOURNAL

As this book shows, I'm a big fan of journaling. It's a great way to remember any event in your life, regardless of whether it involves the possibility of toenails falling off. But the story of threatened toenails deserves to be chronicled in detail. Sometimes when you are actually living through an important time in your life it seems impossible that you will ever not remember exactly what happened. And then menopause kicks in. And then you are having trouble even remembering what kind of Pop-Tarts you prefer. So keep a journal, or a blog, even if you are only able to muster up the energy to scrawl, "Oh, so sore. Even hand muscles hurt. Need full body transplant." Someday, you'll enjoy reading your scribbles, and what better way to remember a story than to read about it all over again?

Where to get it: As luck would have it, you'll find several journal pages conveniently located at the back of this very book. (I know, it's like I designed it that way or something.) If those pages don't offer enough space for your many stories of pulled muscles and dehydration, you can find a decent journal at any bookstore. They come in all shapes and sizes, just like the thoughts you'll put in them. If you don't feel like spending money on what amounts to bound paper, buy a notepad at the supermarket along with your Gatorade and aspirin. Then, when you're adequately hydrated and medicated, you can write a stellar journal entry. If you are more comfortable with a keyboard than a pen, you can finally start that blog you've been meaning to set up. Most are free to create, and they also allow you to post pictures and videos.

CAMERA (STILL AND VIDEO)

Take pictures, lots of them. Be the annoying person who always makes everyone "Pose and look candid!" Pictures are the easiest way to remember your training and see how far you've come. "Can you *believe* I actually thought that top looked cute? My god, I was such an amateur."

I also recommend a video camera. I don't recommend buying one if you don't already have one, but I'm sure you know someone who will let you borrow one. In addition to my written journals, I kept video journals of my training. I'd set up the camera and ramble on about my running escapades. And I'd take the camera out on runs and get footage of my fellow runners. I might be a sucker for a digital memory, but watching those videos instantly takes me back to those training months and reminds me exactly what I was thinking at the time. Most important, it offers video proof that my ab muscles were, for a brief moment in time, actually defined. It was a beautiful moment in time.

Where to get it: Depending on what you choose, cameras can be purchased at the grocery store or at a local electronics store. I say go with a nice disposable one, just in case you accidentally drop it in a water fountain while you're running. (My scientific study shows that you will be considerably less likely to kick said water fountain if the camera is of the disposable variety, instead of the expensive digital model.)

If you don't own a video camera, ask to borrow one once a week to make your home movies. This request might alarm your friends enough that they simply hand over the camera and ask that you not give any further details.

PEOPLE

My final recommendation cannot be purchased at the running store. (Unless you have *a lot* of money. And questionable morals.) I recommend surrounding yourself with great people during your training. Try to find at least one other person to go through this hell with you. He or she will provide you with more support than a sports bra ever could. (In a figurative sense, of course. Unless you are *very* close with your running buddy.)

Your running buddies don't even need to run with you. But they do need to bitch with you. I personally hate running with people, but I absolutely *love* bitching with them. So I run alone and bond with running buddies afterward, comparing our various aches and pains.

Running buddies not only give you people to vent with, they also help keep you honest. They'll call if they don't see you out at the runs. They'll call to see how your run went. They'll call to see if you want to go run. Basically, they'll just keep calling. And you can either change your phone number or just show up and do the damn running.

Plus, just about every good (or bad or ugly) experience in life is better if you have someone to share it with, someone you can call twenty-five years from now and be like, "Remember how much that sucked?" Like you, they'll remember that all the running and sweating and chafing really, really sucked. Like you, they'll also remember that all the laughing and the finish lines and the friendships formed from a common goal were pretty friggin' cool.

● ● ●

HAPPY TRAILS

All these accessories are important to a successful running endeavor. Check out Appendix A (page 225) for a checklist of the items covered in this chapter.

But most important, become comfortable with them in your early weeks. By the time you hit your high mileage, you shouldn't be worrying if your shoes fit right or if your sports bra is too tight or if the cord from your Walkman drives you *insane* when it flaps about. By dealing with your accessories early, you will be free to concentrate on your excruciating pain and overwhelming sense of dread in your higher mileage.

Journal Entry: **WEEK 7**
The Horrors of Short Shorts

It's Week 7. Can you just feel the excitement? I know I can. This week wasn't nearly as fun as last week. That's because I started running again this week. And we all know that running never leads to good times. But I've found that it often leads to food. And that's fun.

The food is most commonly found at the end of organized "event" types of runs. In addition to food, organized runs include numbers that you pin to yourself, people with megaphones yelling motivating tidbits, and, best of all, very excited runners. No matter how ridiculously early it is, these runners are excited to be there. They're moving, they're stretching, they're chatting, they're laughing. They're apparently unaware that it's a Saturday and not past noon. I don't break the news to them because I've made it a rule not to speak that early in the morning. Some of

›››

>>>

these runners are so excited that they actually run to the run. Chipper Jen said that they do this to warm up. I told her that's what the first mile is for.

As the big race gets ready to start, everyone crams together near the start line as though we're about to be released from a high-security prison or are waiting outside a Krispy Kreme that's handing out free doughnuts. I try to visualize the latter, because the excitement of a free doughnut is enough to carry me through a good mile and a half. When the obnoxiously loud bullhorn goes off, the runners begin to move very, very slowly. I cherish this moment. For this is the only moment in which I'm keeping pace with the seven-minute-mile runners. This moment only lasts about thirty seconds; then I'm once again left in the dust by all the runners . . . and two-thirds of the walkers as well.

You think I'm kidding. I'm not. I'm one of the slowest runners you'll ever see. But I'm okay with that. I've found a pace at which I can run eleven miles and not die. That's a good pace for me. There's one thing wrong with it, though. When you're running a pace similar to that of an eighty-year-old asthmatic woman with a wooden leg, pretty much everyone else who is running or walking or riding a bike will pass you. I'm okay with being passed. What I have difficulty with is the number of asses I see as I'm being passed.

The short shorts that runners wear were clearly invented by a very fast runner, a person always at the front who never had to see what the short-shorts runners looked like from behind. Now, I wear spandex while running, which is far from being a pleasant sight. But at least spandex sorta holds things in place. With short shorts, everything is free to

>>>

>>>

wiggle and wobble about. They allow asses to run amok really.

This must be stopped, if not for me, then for the sake of the poor children and wild animals who happen by just as a pair of short shorts comes jiggling down the road. (If we could please pass this anti-ass memo on to bike riders as well, that would be great. People, when you're riding a bike you are bent over to the point that your butt is actually higher than your head. This is not a flattering position, ever. Must we combine short shorts with this already harmful visual? I beg of you to please put an end to this eye-burning trend.)

I don't know about you, but watching people's butts bounce around for miles always makes me hungry. So thank the lord there's food at the end of these event races. There are also quite a few people yelling "Good job!" and offering high-fives. I usually can't give high-fives because I've already filled my arms with heaps of food being handed out. There's fruit and smoothies and sandwiches and even ice cream. It's like Christmas morning, really. Well, it's what Christmas morning would be like if Santa made you run for three hours before giving you any presents.

CHAPTER *four*
The Training

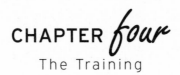

It's important to realize from the start that running is not a competitive sport. The only person you're really competing against is yourself, and you have to like the odds on that. The fastest way to grow frustrated with your training prowess, or lack thereof, is to compare yourself with other runners. Unless you were born in Kenya, you're not going to win a marathon any time soon.

So with that dream shattered, let's concentrate on the whole I'd-prefer-to-not-end-up-in-a-hospital-following-my-attempt-to-finish-a-marathon thing. Avoiding the hospital depends heavily on whether you properly train your poor, unsuspecting body to run a marathon. What follows are some ways to adequately warn that body of yours.

THE STRATEGY

Helping your body endure running long distances is very important. There are as many running strategies as there are runners; everyone has their own unique way of tackling their 26.2. I personally tried about ten different strategies throughout my training, desperately hoping I'd hit on the one that would instantly turn me into a svelte, mobile runner with a zest for ten-minute miles. Sadly, it turns out I might have needed to try out eleven different strategies, because I never quite found the one that turned me into the fantabulous athlete I was aiming to become.

Unless you have an extensive history of running and/or Kenyan heritage, I recommend you experiment with various run/walk combinations during your training. A famous guy named Jeff Galloway revolutionized the marathon world by suggesting that maybe it's okay to walk a little instead of running nonstop for the entire 26.2 miles. I worry about the collective intelligence of the marathon world if this guy was really the first person to think this up; but he's the one credited with introducing common sense to the running world. Quite an honor indeed.

You can implement Jeff's run/walk program in countless ways (I implemented ten ways myself), and each long run offers you the chance to experiment with what works best for you. Some runners use their watches to time running and walking, walking one minute for every five minutes they run, or two minutes for every ten minutes. They do this throughout long runs, providing a break for their bodies at regular intervals. Personally, I found that this strategy did not work well at all with my efforts to remain sane. If you're looking for a way to make your run seem absolutely endless, check your watch. Do it now. Tell yourself that something wonderful will happen in two minutes, then try not to look at said watch every three seconds to see if you're closer to that wonderful thing happening. You see how this could become an issue on a three-hour run.

The strategy I settled on didn't involve a watch; it involved mile markers that seemed to grow farther apart the farther I ran. I'd run a mile and then walk for a minute, then run a mile and walk a minute, etc. Toward the end of my training, when my knee began to take leave of my body, I'd also stop to do a knee-preserving stretch every mile. This routine worked better than the timing method because I was only looking out for the next mile marker. I didn't have to consult a watch that purposely ran slower the more I anticipated my walking time.

One thing I noticed about my run/walk routine was that walking seemed to do more harm than good toward the end of super-long runs. By that time my poor body was hanging on for dear life; and every time I stopped to walk, my muscles believed we were finally done with this ridiculous movement and they all tightened up at the same time to celebrate. This would make my walking slightly uncomfortable and my return to running even more uncomfortable. To prevent this discomfort, I merely slowed my pace at mile markers, but didn't completely stop running, allowing myself a little rest without giving my poor muscles any false hope. Many people I know swear by Galloway's method and do every walk break. These people's muscles are much more cooperative than mine. If you can convince your body to start running again after a walk break at Mile 23 then more power to you.

I'm not exaggerating when I say I tried at least ten different run/walk strategies during my training; you too may end up experimenting with that many. Just remember that long-distance running involves ups and downs, both figuratively and literally. You'll reach points in your higher mileage when things start to feel very unpleasant. This isn't your strategy failing; it's your body becoming annoyed and your mind trying to convince you it's time to stop and take up a more sensible hobby, such as needlepoint. You will need a specific strategy to deal with these times as well, because they will arise more than once during your marathon. Pushing through these times will give you confidence to push through them during your marathon.

Like anything in your training, the goal is to find a workable strategy and use it so much that your body gets used to it. This is what training is all about, slowly tricking your body into believing that it's a marathon runner.

Journal Entry: WEEK 4
Cheetos and a Nap

I figured out how many miles I've run in the past month. The total came to sixty-one miles. *Sixty-one miles.* What the . . . ? If you do the math, you realize it's too much friggin' running. Nine of those miles came all at once last weekend. Yes, I ran nine consecutive miles. In the morning. On a holiday. Something has gone terribly wrong with my life plan. A friend of mine, Erika, was visiting from out of town and decided to join Chipper Jen and me for our nine-mile run. I don't know about you, but every time I'm visiting friends and family I always like to get in a good nine-mile run. I think I need new, less-motivated friends.

With the addition of a third runner, Jen became extra chipper. She finally had someone to talk to. As I've mentioned, I do not enjoy anything when I run. There will be no talking, there will be no pointing out of good-looking people, there will be no smiling and/or laughing. There will only be me listening to my radio and trying very hard to keep my kneecaps from dislocating. Apparently Erika's kneecaps can be left unattended, which allowed her plenty of time to converse with Jen. I can't tell you what they talked about because: (1) I can't hear over my radio music; and (2) I can't hear from a hundred yards away. That's about how far in front of me the two little chitchatters

>>>

>>>

were. Yes, they ditched me. Very sad. I would have cried, but it would have consumed too much of my valuable fluids.

I think they were trying to motivate me to move faster by setting a faster pace and forcing me to keep up with them—a good idea in theory. But that idea doesn't work well with me. I'm not one who particularly cares what anyone else is doing. If everyone else is running faster than me, that's great for them. I'm fine doing my own thing at the back of the pack. This isn't the best mentality when training for a marathon, but over the years it's done me more good than harm. Peer pressure has never been a big issue for me. "Hey, everyone's smoking pot, you should too." "No thanks, I'm fine just eating a bag of Cheetos and taking a nap; I'll skip the smoking-out part."

Coincidently, Jen and I came across a couple of potheads during a recent run along the river. Before I tell you about them, I'll tell you a little about my hearing. Because there's very little to tell about my hearing. Basically I have none. I've always been hard of hearing, and a few years ago I got hearing aids. I call them "my ears." They cost about as much as you'd pay to have new ears surgically put on your head. I take them out when I run because I don't think sweat is good for computer chips. Then I put on my headphones. And, well, then Dawn is pretty much deaf to the world.

So we're running along the river one day and I smell marijuana. I look at Jen, who has her nose up in the air like a police dog and a slight frown on her face. So, either she smells it too, or she's trying to do long division in her head. As we come around a corner we see two boys standing down by the river smoking pot. When they see us, they frantically pretend to examine

>>>

their bikes, their shoes, the trees, in a valiant but un-successful effort to look drug-free. I found this amus-ing; so I said, in what I thought was a library voice, "Look at those two guys, they're smoking pot, they're trying to hide it." Unfortunately, because of my lack of hearing and my blaring radio, the statement came out loud enough for the boys, the bikes, the shoes, all the trees, and some fellow runners to hear, "LOOK AT THOSE TWO GUYS. THEY'RE SMOKING POT, THEY'RE TRYING TO HIDE IT!" Oops.

Back at my nine-mile run, as I watched Erika and Jen bounce off in the distance, I wondered if I could trade my two motivated friends for a couple of potheads. I bet potheads don't run sixty-one miles a month. And I could really use some Cheetos and a nap.

THE PACE

Pace is another issue you'll need to experiment with. The watch I threw to the ground in frustration during the run/walk timing fiasco actually came in handy when I wanted to figure out how slowly I was running. Everyone finds a pace that allows them to comfortably run for miles and miles when there's no hope of public transportation coming to save them. Once you find that pace you'll probably hover around it for most of your training. It may go up or down, depending on circumstances (e.g., injuries and newfound superhuman running powers); but on the whole, once you find your pace you're going to want to stay near it, since that's what's going to allow you to see the higher miles.

I was told that the best way to find your pace is to run at a speed at which you can carry on a conversation. My trainers actual-ly call it a "conversational pace." I can make no personal validation of its effectiveness because, as I am hearing-impaired and always run without my hearing aids, conversations are kinda out of the question for me. Occasionally, in an effort to be a good friend and running buddy, I pretend to listen to runners chat while we bounce along, but I've never tested out the talking-while-running thing, as I wouldn't have any idea what the hell the other person was saying. On the upside, I have a reputation for being a very good listener.

The point of the "conversational pace" is to keep you from pushing so hard that you run out of energy for later miles. If you want to push yourself to run a faster mile, I'd recommend doing it on the shorter runs, when you won't be needing your energy reserves or any of those silly conversations.

THE STRETCHING

Before I started training, I never in my life figured out the purpose of stretching. I'd grown up playing sports, but I'd usually just go through the motions of stretching and never actually feel anything stretching at all. This changed when I started running. In addition to becoming very aware of all my leg muscles whether I was running or not, I began to feel my muscles actually stretch when I stretched. Who knew?

There are a million different stretches you can do to make you a flexible running machine. People have written entire books *just about stretching*. I find that slightly intimidating, since I'm trying to summarize stretching in a paragraph or two. I must be missing something, because my total time stretching usually maxes out at a few minutes.

I learned about stretching not from a book, but from random runners I happened by on my training runs. I will now share all that I learned about stretching over the course of my training. Think of it as the Cliff's Notes guide to stretching:

Stretching is a very important part of your running routine, and it's important that it be done correctly. First, you don't need to stretch much before your run. It's recommended that you warm your muscles up a little before doing any major stretching. This means that you can use your first mile or two as a slow alert to your muscles that they're now becoming part of an active lifestyle. After the muscles have time to wake up and join the run already in progress, you can stop and stretch out the very disgruntled body parts. Some people (insane people) actually run a mile or two to warm up before stretching and *before* even *starting* their run. I would always see these people *running to the runs* and think that there had to be something mentally wrong with them. That's like getting a pap smear before your annual gyno visit, just 'cause you want to get ready. Like I said, these people have mental issues.

In addition to stretching during your run, it is recommended that you stretch a little after your run. This will help your body move comfortably from running mode back to comatose mode by reducing the uncomfortable all-muscles-are-tightening-up-to-celebrate-the-end-of-the-run mode. Some people (the insane ones I mentioned earlier) actually choose to do their postrun stretches and then continue their warm-down with another one- or two-mile jog. I hate to make two gynecological analogies in the course of two paragraphs, so I leave it to you to figure out what I think about running after a run is over.

Stretching Help

SOME COMMON RUNNING STRETCHES AND WHAT THEY MOST CLOSELY RESEMBLE IN YOUR PRE-MARATHON LIFE.

Stretches are hard to explain, so I thought I'd draw you some pictures. But, I don't draw too well. So, please excuse the poor artistry and instead concentrate on the extremely helpful stretching guide. Also, ignore the fact that the stick-figure Stretcher Guy seems to be wearing mittens. Fingers are hard to draw. Don't wear mittens while stretching. You will look silly. Unfortunately, the hat with the holes is not an artistic creation; it's actually what your running hat will look like. So you might as well wear the mittens, 'cause you're already gonna look silly.

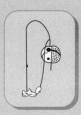

1. RUNNING STRETCH

Bend over and touch your toes (or as close as you can get to your toes) and stretch out your hamstrings.

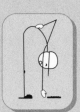

1. *NON* ∧ RUNNER LIFE

You've been doing this stretch for years, every time you drop the remote and have to bend over and pick it up. (If you have children who are old enough to pick it up for you, you might have to think way back to remember how to do this stretch.)

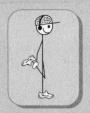

2. RUNNING STRETCH

Pull your ankle up toward your butt keeping your knees together and hips aligned, and stretch out your quadriceps.

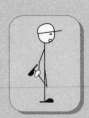

2. NON RUNNER LIFE

You know how sometimes when you get up to greet the pizza delivery guy, you accidentally ram your foot into an inconveniently placed end table? The quad stretch is a lot like the "Oh my god that hurts" stretch you do until your toe stops throbbing.

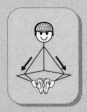

3. RUNNING STRETCH

Sit with the bottoms of your feet touching and your knees out to their sides. Put your elbows on your knees and slowly push them down. This will stretch your groin.

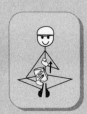

3. NON RUNNER LIFE

I'm imagining you have a lot of different reference points for this stretch, seeing how it involves sitting on the ground. I picked my favorite pre-marathon sitting stretch—the ever-popular Chip Lift.

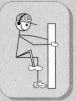

4. RUNNING STRETCH

This one is a bit complicated, but it really helped my poor IT band (a band that runs from hip to knee). The IT band can cause many a problem, so try out this stretch. Basically you cross your legs as you would while sitting in a chair, and then, holding on to a tree or post, sit down like you're in a chair. Do this slowly and you will feel the stretch.

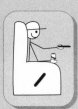

4. *NON* RUNNER LIFE

You've done this stretch tons of times, but have actually been sitting in a chair while doing it. In that version, you don't quite feel the burn.

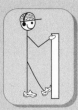

5. RUNNING STRETCH

Find a wall or a tree or a person who isn't in a hurry and put your toes up against it/him/her while leaving your heel on the ground. This will stretch out your calves.

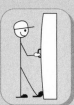

5. *NON* RUNNER LIFE

You know when you open the freezer to get some ice for your soda and the freezer door gets a little stuck and you have to hold the fridge side of the door with your foot while you pull the freezer open? This stretch is similar to that. Except that after you're done, you get heatstroke instead of a cool beverage.

THE ROUTE

You have numerous options when it comes to places where you can run. Each has its own set of pros and cons, and each one will probably end up with your footprint on it by the end of your training.

A likely option is the local running track, often found at high schools and colleges, because apparently those young'uns sure do love to run. Tracks are a good place to run because the track itself is usually made of material that's a lot more friendly to your knees than surfaces you'll find in other locations. Also, if you're a night runner (not to be confused with Knight Rider—what I wouldn't have given for that talking car around Mile 20 of my marathon), it's sometimes difficult to find outdoor running areas that don't make you wonder exactly how many strange people are lurking in the shadows waiting to attack. Tracks are usually well lit and can provide a safe place for you to get in a few miles. But if you're doing anything over a few miles, you are probably not going to be able to take the tediousness of having to run around that damn track four times just to log one mile.

If you want a little more variety, find a nearby park that has a jogging trail or perhaps just a sidewalk that circles the perimeter. The trails are often full of other runners, and the park itself is usually full of people doing park things. These people and their park things can offer some visual distractions from the physical insanity in which you're participating. Like the track, however, park trails often only work for lower mileage, not double-digit runs. They're entertaining, yes, but after nine miles you'll be saying, "You all are having the single most boring barbeque in the history of outdoor cooking; let's liven things up a bit people!"

When you set off on your long runs, you'll usually want to do so on a running trail of some sort. These can usually be found near a river, although I have no idea why. I've always found it to be cruelly ironic how thirsty and hot I feel while running next to a rushing stream of water. But you really can't beat the open, endless miles a good running trail provides. When I tackled my long runs, I'd run half the distance, then turn around and run the other half back in. I'm convinced these trails are the only reason I completed any long runs. The trails wound through wooded areas far away from roads of any kind, leaving running (or moving, at least) as my only viable option for ever reentering society. If I had had a viable option that didn't involve running past Mile 9, I can't say for sure that I would have ever completed my training.

Running trails often have both asphalt and dirt trails, the latter preferred by countless runners trying to preserve their poor knees. Although you'll probably be running your marathon on asphalt, try to train on softer, less jarring surfaces. This will help not just your knees but countless other joints that absorb the jolting shock of your feet pounding against the pavement or dirt or track.

Sometimes weather or time of day doesn't allow you the option of running outside. In that case, you can always rely on the handy treadmill. I don't recommend them for anything above five miles, only because I know how tremendously boring they can be. Also, unlike the running trail, the treadmill provides *nothing* but options for stopping. Now, I know you are a strong-willed, undeterred wall of focus when you run, but dammit if that little STOP button doesn't wear you down after awhile.

THE LIQUIDS

Let me introduce you to liquids. The two of you are going to be spending a lot of time together. Hydration, hydration, hydration. Very important in the non-passing-out efforts of long-distance runners. Keeping your body hydrated before, during, and after a run will keep you healthy and a little happier out there on that trail.

Before you even start your run, think about hydration. And, keep thinking about it throughout your training. (Go ahead, I'll wait while you think about it a moment.) You need to make sure your body is always properly hydrated. Apparently the way to gauge whether you're taking in enough water is to look at your urine. (Go ahead, I'll wait.) Your urine should be relatively clear or flourescent if you're taking vitamins; if it's darker, then you failed the urine test and need to drink more liquids and try again later. It is also recommended that you drink water an hour or two before your run so you have some reserves when you hit the course.

It is typically recommended you drink water—from six to twelve ounces—every fifteen minutes during longer runs. Do this throughout the entire run, not just when you feel thirsty. Thirst is not a signal that you need hydration (I know—this is just one more example why I should have paid attention in science class). By the time you experience thirst, IT'S TOO LATE! Well, it's not quite that dramatic, but I thought the caps might scare you into proper hydration. Basically, if you wait till you're thirsty, you're going to be doing some major catch-up, which means bad news for your run.

Here's the fun part. Although hydration is very important, *too much* water can actually hurt you. Who understands science at all?

Overdrinking can cause this thing called hyponatremia, and with effects like comas, seizures, and death, it doesn't sound like a fun way to end a run. So how do you dodge death by dehydration and death by overhydration? Hop on the scale, of course.

Weigh yourself before and after a run to determine how much weight you've lost. This weight loss is most likely water (although you can go ahead and believe it's that chocolate cake you ate last night). Add the amount of weight you lost to the amount of water you took in while you were running and the result of the equation will be the total amount of water your body used during your run. In future runs of similar time frames you'll need to be conscious of this water intake and make an effort to drink enough throughout your run to keep the same amount of fluids going into your body as you know are being sweated out.

As far as your choices for hydration, sports drinks are recommended for longer runs when your body needs carbohydrates, electrolytes, and sodium. What combination of sports drinks and water you choose is up to you. Personally, I carried my sports drink on me during my training and still often stopped at water fountains. On race day you can make use of aid stations that will have both water and sports drinks available for you.

After you finish your run, you're not done with hydration. It's recommended you drink two cups of water for every pound you lost during your run, and it's important to stay hydrated well after you have completed your allotted sweating for the day. I've been told to wait until I started urinating before I started rehydrating after my run, to avoid the dreaded overhydration, so I will pass this piece of advice to you. "I've got to pee! Break out the beverages!"

THE FOOD

It's all about the carbs, baby. The world of running is an anti-Atkins world, and that makes it not such a bad world after all. Carbohydrates provide important fuel for anyone doing intense physical training. Therefore you're allowed to go carb-happy for the sake of your overall health and well-being. It's a miracle, really.

Carbs should account for 60 to 70 percent of your total daily calories while you are training. They can be found in all sorts of fun stuff like bread, pasta, rice, fruit, vegetables, and low-fat dairy foods. If you are wondering about a food's carb content, you can usually find it on the nutrition label. Be careful not to accidentally pick up one of those low-carb concoctions that may taste carb-tastic, but is in fact just another product of the carb-free craze that's swept the nation in various manifestations through the years.

Protein is the next major thing on your diet list. It helps muscles grow and repair themselves. However, in our anti-Atkins world, protein is not as important as carbs and therefore should only account for 12 to 15 percent of your daily caloric intake. Protein can be found in meat, fish, chicken, eggs, tofu, and nuts, all of which sound like the ingredients for a very creative meatloaf.

As much as it pains me to admit, a proper marathon diet is low in fat. Just take comfort in your carbs when the whole low-fat thing comes up.

Journal Entry: WEEK 11
A Big Day

I'm supposed to run eighteen miles this weekend. In a row. So there's a good possibility that this may be the last journal entry I ever write. In the off chance I do survive, it could be sometime next year before I complete eighteen miles, if you combine my running speed with my tendency to nap between miles. Any way you look at it, the odds of a journal entry any time soon are not good.

The most exciting thing that's happened to me since I started training has to be the fact that yesterday Chipper Jen actually uttered the words, "I hate running." It was quite a moment indeed. Those words nearly brought a tear to my eye. They were spoken shortly after the statement, "In the past two weeks I drank myself silly eight times and ran no times." You see, little Chipper has been away on a cruise and is having trouble adjusting to life here on dry land. "I'm still on cruise-time," she kept saying. The cruise was to Mexico, so I'm not quite sure where different time zones come into play. But details are unimportant. The important thing is, *Jen hated running yesterday!!!* Yes, that deserves *three* exclamation points, and I'm not one to just throw exclamation points around haphazardly. It's really that exciting to me. Less exciting is the fact that a hungover, out-of-shape Jen is feeling about the same as a sober, buffed-up Dawn. But again, details are not important.

And speaking of a sober, buffed-up Dawn, she still hasn't lost a pound. Not even one. After running 185 miles in three months. Nothin'. How is it even scientifically possible to lose no weight after 185 miles? I

>>>

>>>

think it's my body's revenge for all this activity. "You can make me get up early, you can make me run in circles, and you can make me eat PowerBars. But I'll be damned if I'm gonna let go of even one pound. Weight loss may encourage post-marathon exercising, and that simply cannot and will not happen."

Friends of mine have implied that perhaps I'm not losing weight because I'm gaining so much muscle. I think they might have a point. I'm beginning to see noticeable differences in my body, most noticeably in my muscles, most noticeably that I seem to have some now. It's a bit weird. I've never been one to notice my body at all. I always look the same every time I look in the mirror, no matter if my weight has gone up or down. I'm one of those people who only knows what she looks like when she sees a picture of herself. And even then it's usually a picture from years ago and I exclaim, "Why didn't anyone tell me I was so skinny?! I would have made a note to enjoy it more!"

Now I am forcing myself to note the appearance of muscles on my body because I fear they may disappear the minute I stop running. Someday I want to be able to say to the grandkids, "Come sit on Grandma's lap so she can tell you a story about when she had ab muscles. They were fantastic." And the grandkids will say, "Where are the ab muscles now, Grandma?" To which I'll reply, in a cautionary tone, "I lost them shortly after I finished my marathon, during an unfortunate incident involving four bags of Cheetos, my recliner, and a Chinese restaurant with free delivery until midnight."

So then, as you can see, a lot of noteworthy things are happening here. We've got Jen hating running and me having ab muscles. Maybe I should stock up on canned goods. The end may be near.

SORTA LIQUID/SORTA FOOD

The wonder that is GU is difficult to categorize. Calling it a food would be an insult to culinary arts; but calling it a liquid would be a stretch. What we do know about GU and other gel-type, energy-rich products is that they provide us with a way to take in calories and other important things while we're running and don't have time to stop for a meal.

As you start to get up into your higher mileage, you'll need to start putting calories and carbs into your body to keep up with the insane amount of calories you're burning. GU and similar products provide a quick and easy means to get those calories your body needs. It's recommended you take in one GU packet (a hundred calories) every forty-five minutes to an hour while you're training. Wash it down with water, not a sports drink.

In my experience, I usually started the GU a little later in my run, but tried to remember it before I was feeling the effects of the long run. By the time you start feeling like you might need GU, you'll again be playing catch-up. Usually you won't get caught up and you will end up feeling very sluggish as you try to finish the run. Well, even more sluggish than you do any other time throughout the run.

CROSS-TRAINING

To help your body survive the rigors of marathon training, you need to do some physical activity other than just running for five months straight. Cross-training allows you to continue exercising, even on days when you aren't running, and gives your poor joints a moment of nonjarring physical activity. When choosing an activity, keep three words in mind: exercise without impact.

Popular cross-training activities include swimming, bicycling, weight lifting, stair-climbing, rowing, and other low-impact workouts. I chose swimming. My knees were in bad shape throughout my training and swimming was calming to my ravaged joints. It gave me the opportunity to work my upper body a little. Plus, I've never looked better in a swimsuit, so I thought I might as well be in a pool when I was showing off this revelation.

It's important to remember that cross-training is not a substitute for running and is never meant to be done on days allotted for rest. This seems obvious to me, but you'll find some exercise-happy people swimming laps on their "rest day" because they think they're just supposed to be resting from running. People, the word "rest" will not appear often during your months of training, so when it does, do not waste even a second of it flexing even one single muscle.

THE GOAL

The most important goal of your training is to survive it and arrive at your marathon in one functioning piece. The other goal is to have trained well enough to continue your survival streak through the end of the marathon. As you work your way through training, you'll find various things that do and do not work for you. Use the months leading up to the marathon to figure out what works for you as a runner and as a person who wishes to cross the finish line without needing to be resuscitated along the course.

By the time you get to the start line of your marathon, you should have a clear idea of how you intend to tackle the 26.2 miles that lie ahead. The fact that there are 26.2 miles ahead will worry you a little, but that worry shouldn't be the result of a lack of preparation. (That worry should probably come as a result of all the people who will be finishing the marathon before you reach the halfway point.) In your months of training you'll have plenty of time to figure out important things such as what running pace you prefer, what meals agree with your stomach before a run, and what running shorts make your ass look best. You know, all the important things.

Once you've figured out these things through trial and error ("Girl, those shorts are just not doing your booty any justice at all"), do not veer away from them on marathon day. I repeat, DO NOT. I repeat because it was repeated to me in all caps repeatedly. Apparently very bad things will happen if you veer away from the habits your body has grown comfortable with (or at least tolerant of) during training.

Also, please remember that in order to *finish* your marathon, you actually have to *start* it. That means you need to survive the training, and that means that the training is not a place to kill yourself in an effort to surpass those pesky Serious Runners. Listen to your body throughout your training. If it's feeling Kenyan-esque, then by all means, push yourself to your full champion potential. But if at any time you feel more Homer Simpson-esque, don't beat yourself up for slowing down a little and preserving your fragile body for the sake of longevity. Burnout is one of the top reasons people end up dropping out of marathon training. They start with a flash of brilliance and determination and end when the luster and excitement wear off. (In my case, the luster wore off 3.2 seconds after I bought my first pair of shoes and then realized I actually had to *run* while wearing them.) So remember that your training, just like the marathon itself, is an endurance event.

Take it slow and steady, and you'll find that not only are you able to endure it, but you can thrive as well.

Here is space for you to jot down some of the highs and lows of your training. It will be fun to look back at how far you've come and how far you thought you'd come when you really had no idea how far you still had to go.

MILES RAN: _____

STRATEGY: _____

_____

PACE: _____

RESULT: _____

_____

MILES RAN: _____

STRATEGY: _____

_____

PACE: _____

RESULT: _____

_____

MILES RAN: _____

STRATEGY: _____

_____

PACE: _____

RESULT: _____

_____

MILES RAN: _____

STRATEGY: _____

_____

PACE: _____

RESULT: _____

_____

MILES RAN: _____

STRATEGY: _____

_____

PACE: _____

RESULT: _____

_____

MILES RAN: _____

STRATEGY: _____

_____

PACE: _____

RESULT: _____

_____

MILES RAN: _____

STRATEGY: _____

_____

PACE: _____

RESULT: _____

_____

Journal Entry: WEEK 12
Graduation

The park where I frequently run is just about the cutest park ever. Its cuteness supplies me with endless visual distractions while I run: people playing Frisbee, people playing tennis, people huddled near the bushes drinking out of paper bags. In addition to being a meeting area for people looking for individual fun, the park is a favorite location for many community classes, like tai chi and outdoor painting.

The most entertaining of these classes meets every Tuesday and Thursday—dog obedience class. Early in my training, the dogs were just beginning their training too. As I ran around the park, mile after mile, I loved watching the owners attempting to train their dogs and the dogs attempting to chase every runner in the park. At least twice a night, a dog would escape its owner and gleefully start running alongside some unsuspecting jogger. The jogger would either greet the dog with a smile or freak the hell out because they thought they were being attacked by a rabid canine. Guess which response I enjoyed more.

As the weeks have gone by, the class has became calmer and quieter (much to my disappointment). But every once in a while, a dog goes AWOL and rebels against all the proper behavior it's been taught. It is those problem students that keep me going. There is always the hope of someone getting attacked by an obedience school dropout.

Last Tuesday, as I jogged by the class site, I saw tables with food and beverages set up instead of the normal circle of dogs and owners. I wondered where the class

>>>

>>>

had been moved to in order to make room for this party. On closer examination, I realized that dogs and owners were at the party. It was a graduation party!

I smiled as I realized that the dogs and I had much in common: We'd taken on quite a challenge these past months. I secretly wished that at the finish of the marathon, I could wear a pointy party hat, just like the ones the dogs were made to wear at their graduation party. But then, I'll be wearing spandex, so I already might exceed my ridiculous-attire quota. A party hat could push it over the edge.

CHAPTER *five*
The Limit

We all have our limits. The maximum we can take (or spend, if we're talking credit cards). But the fact is that we as human beings rarely approach our limits (unless we're talking credit cards again, 'cause we seem to be fine at pushing ourselves past those limits). Things we perceive as personal limits usually just mark the limit of our comfort level, not the limit of any actual ability. It's not until we're challenged that most of us ever know what we are really capable of doing.

We've all heard the story of the mom who was able to muster the strength to lift a whole car off her baby (though I often wonder how the mother allowed her baby to end up *under* the car in the first place). Stories of human strength and triumph remind us that we too might be capable of lifting a car if challenged to do so. But really, how often do car-lifting opportunities present themselves in real life?

That's where your marathon comes in. If challenges aren't presenting themselves to you, sometimes it's best to go seek them out. And your marathon training will be just the car-lifting challenge you've been looking for. (Of course, in the mother/baby/car metaphor, the marathon trainee usually ends up feeling more like the baby than the mom.)

One of the greatest things that will come as a result of your marathon training (besides a new ability to spot and use appropriate peeing locations on a running trail with lightning speed) will be the absolute shattering of what you used to accept as your physical and mental limitations. The first time you look at your training calendar, you'll be overwhelmed by the numbers you see before you. You'll wonder how you'll make it past the first few weeks, let alone all the way to the marathon finish line.

Even after you start training, you'll wonder if your limit might be more Fun Run and less 26.2-Miles-in-a-Row Run. But you will continue to run and you will continue to surprise yourself with your ability to keep running right past those weeks on your training calendar that once seemed so insurmountable. And you'll realize that the only real limitation you ever had was your inability to see what you were actually capable of all along.

For a person like me—one who has honed laziness to an art form—personal limits seem very, very low. But such a person also has that annoying voice in the back of her head constantly reminding her that merely "coasting by" in life isn't an accomplishment. Normally this voice is drowned out by all the noise made by crunching on Cheetos and watching cable TV. But once in a while, the cable goes out and the Cheetos bag is empty. Then such a person is left with an overwhelming sense of fading potential. And if lack of cable and Cheetos isn't enough to inspire change, I just don't know what is.

I decided to train for a marathon because I wanted to know my limits. I wanted to see if I were capable of a physical activity that involved more than reaching *reeeeeally* far for the remote control. As I trained for the marathon, it became apparent that, yes, my limits were much higher than I'd ever expected, but at the same time my threshold for pain remained quite low.

Following my first seven-mile run, I collapsed on the grass near my running trail, hoping that complete lack of movement would help cool the heat now pulsating through my face. All I could do was lay there, listening to my heartbeat and my gasping, rapid breaths. Although I felt like I might die at any moment, I realized that this feeling of exhaustion was exactly the reason I was training for a marathon. I am an able-bodied, young person who, up until that point, had done everything in her power to avoid this sort of exhaustion (because I am also quite intelligent).

But I set out to train for a marathon because I knew there was no physical reason why I shouldn't be able to do it. Sure, it wasn't going to be easy to go from the recliner to running miles at a time. But lying on the grass, wondering if my heart was going to explode, I was able to muster a smile—I knew I had just pushed myself past my perceived limits, limits I had long ago accepted only because I wasn't motivated enough to try to do more.

Although you'll be amazed at the limits you'll exceed, it's also important to distinguish between real limits and those that just seem real because your legs feel like they've turned to Jell-O. There's actually a very thin line between imaginary limits and real limits, and it's important not to cross over that line and into the intensive care unit.

● ● ●

Journal Entry: WEEK 2

The First Three Miles

Two weeks into my training, I ran into someone from my training team. This overly enthusiastic woman overly enthusiastically asked me if she'd see me at the 7 AM team run on Saturday. In my moderately enthusiastic way, I said, "Sure, I'll see you out there."

Riiiiiiight. You see, I don't like mornings, especially weekend mornings. And to be honest, they don't enjoy me too much either. So when I heard that the team runs were going to be taking place at 7 AM on Saturday, I was less than thrilled. But if that was what it was going to take, well then, by golly, that's what I was gonna do. But the odds of me actually getting out of bed at 7 AM on a Saturday are about as good as the odds I'll ever use the phrase "by golly" again in my life. So, needless to say, when 7 AM rolled around on Saturday, I had a slight change of heart. I like to think of it as a change of logic really. It went something like this: *I hate mornings and I hate running. So why on earth would I feel the need to combine the two for what will surely be an unhappy union? Why not wait until a more suitable hour, like say, noon, to do the horrible moving of my body?*

So that's what I did. I slept until a more humane time and then I got up and ran the required three miles on my own. You think I'm lying don't you? I'm not. I really did run three miles. Was it fun? No. Was it fulfilling? No. But most important, was it 7 AM? Thank the lord, no.

Before I went for my inaugural run, I decided to measure it with my car. I mapped out a route that

>>>

>>>

equaled three miles on my speedometer—leaving from my house and ending at my house—a circle of sorts through downtown. Then I parked my car and ran that route. A couple things went wrong with this plan. First, I live downtown, so the entire three miles was along roads with lots of cars. When running your first major mileage, I do not recommend having car fumes nearby. Because you're going to be gasping for breath. And sucking in car fumes is not nearly as much fun as you'd imagine.

Second, it wasn't morning time anymore. And as much as I disagree with the basic principles of morning, I must hand it to the AM hours—they are nice and cool. The PM hours, not so cool. Of course, before today I'd never really noticed that they weren't cool, because before today I'd never really had occasion to force my heart rate up to that of a sprinting racehorse on speed. That tends to warm things up a bit. As I was running along a busy downtown street, with the sun beating down on me, I slowly started to see why people choose to run in tree-lined parks before the sun has the opportunity to rise directly overhead. *Hmphh.* By the time I got home I feared that death was imminent. Never in my life has my heart beat so fast. And with every beat a new spurt of sweat seemed to jump off my face. Which seemed weird, 'cause my face was so hot I would've thought that all the sweat would have evaporated on contact. But it didn't. It continued to flow, as if from some unlimited sweat reserve that hasn't been tapped since that one time when I was ten and decided that a push-pop was worth chasing the ice cream man for two blocks.

I didn't think it was possible, but I actually got hotter once I stopped running. It seemed every ounce of my blood had rushed to my face and was screaming with

>>>

>>>

every pulse, *Let me out. Let me out. So hot in here. Boiling up.* The second I got home I went straight to my kitchen and laid facedown on the floor. My face needed to be next to something cool, and I needed to no longer be vertical, so the tile in the kitchen seemed like a great way to bring all my needs together. It felt like hours that I lay there, my body bouncing with every heartbeat, trying so hard to right the many, many wrongs that were going on. I tried to figure out how to drink water while facedown on the floor. I ended up nearly drowning myself by pouring water near my mouth and trying to suck it in before it fell to the tile. When I realized that a marathon is twenty-three more miles than I just ran, I tried to end my misery by pouring the whole bottle of water on my face.

As you can see, the training is going really well so far.

IMAGINARY LIMITS

1. The word *can't*

I don't mean to get all Motivational Speaker on you, but the word *can't* is a complete waste of breath. It's also one of the most incorrectly used words in the dictionary. Frankly, there aren't many things in this life you can't do. There are a hell of a lot of things you don't *want* to do, and that's fine; but never confuse the two words. Your training goal is to finish the marathon. There are many ways to do this: You can run the entire route; you can walk the entire route; or you can run some and walk some. And believe me, by using one of those options you can successfully complete your training.

So if while you train you begin to feel the word *can't* making its way to your lips, pinch those lips closed immediately and remember that *can't* is not a valid limit. Yes, it may be ridiculously difficult at times to muster the energy to keep trucking, and it may seem easier to simply chalk it up to your physical limitations than to keep pushing forward. But those are the times you have to be creative and figure out ways—any way—to get yourself back on the running trail. Maybe you'll slow down your pace, maybe you'll invite a new friend along to liven things up, maybe you'll chase an ice cream truck around your neighborhood. Whatever it takes.

One of the most effective ways to stay motivated is to constantly remind yourself that this can be done. If you honestly believe it, you'll be able to push on, even when your body is doubtful. I mean, it worked for the little steam engine in *The Little Engine That Could,* right? So you should be fine. Your caboose is nothing compared with his.

2. Your mind

More than any muscle pulls or rashes or Houdini-like sports bras, your mind may prove to be your biggest obstacle throughout your training. At least that was the case for me, which is saying a lot, because my obstacles were varied and plentiful. Yet my mind posed the greatest threat to my training. I tend to be a glass-half-empty kind of girl, a nearly debilitating mindset when you're trying to tackle long runs and months of training. I became overwhelmed with what lay ahead, whether it was a long run or the entire remaining training schedule.

Henry Ford once said, "Whether you think you can, or you think you can't, you're right." I love that sentiment. It's true about many things in life, but it's 100 percent true when it comes to marathon training. Despite all the physical limitations you'll overcome, you will be forced to deal with even more mental limitations. Your mind will decide whether your training will be successful; if you are mentally convinced you'll succeed, then you'll be able to convince the rest of your body. But if you aren't convinced then that attitude will slowly seep into your physical performance and you will slowly begin to accept limits that are far less than what you are capable of accomplishing.

A negative attitude or dread of All Things Running is not impossible to overcome. First, try to surround yourself with fellow runners who have an upbeat attitude. Some of these people are so damn happy about running you can't help but think that perhaps they have a point. Second, lighten up. Have a sense of humor about your abilities, or lack thereof. Humor can be found pretty much anywhere you look, and it makes any journey that much more enjoyable.

Once you shift your attitude, you'll also notice a shift in what you can do, simply because you now believe you can.

3. Wanting to quit every run after the first two miles

Serious Runners often talk about The Wall they hit as they get into the higher mileage of training or races. This wall is similar to a real wall in that you feel like you've just slammed full-force into a very immovable object. Usually this wall is not the race-ender it seems; it's merely another perceived limitation you need to run through.

Proving once again that I'm not a Serious Runner, I usually hit my wall at about Mile 2 of every run. For some reason, Mile 2 consistently proved to be nearly insurmountable. I wanted to stop running, I wanted to go home, I wanted to know why I was having these feelings before I'd even managed to break a sweat. There was no real physical reason for my Mile 2 wall, but I would push through it and then I was able to fall into a rhythm for the remainder of the run.

Prior to my training, when I had occasion to run (usually away from something very frightening or toward something very enticing), I always stopped when I hit that Mile 2 wall (actually it was more like a Mile .2 wall). It usually only happened once a year during PE, and then only if I had a female teacher who wasn't buying my I-can't-run-today-I-have-*female*-problems excuse. Female problems or not, I stopped running when I hit my wall because it felt like a limit. Once I started training, I was alarmed to meet my limit at Mile 2 and wondered if the remaining twenty-four miles of the marathon were important. Maybe I could just keep doing two miles over and over again throughout my training. Then one day I kept running past the Mile 2 wall and was surprised when I did not die as a result. I realized, almost in awe, that my wall was nothing but an illusion, my mind's way of nipping any running silliness in the bud before things got out of hand. Imagine all the places I could have run throughout the years!

Everyone has a different time during their run when they feel more sluggish and less excited about their choice of pastimes. But if you keep running through that feeling, eventually it will fade away into an acceptance and perhaps even a slight enjoyment. You might even get to that "Runner's High" the Serious Runners always talk about, which is a hell of a lot better than the "Runner's Bleh" you feel when you hit the wall. The first time you experience those endorphins kick in, you'll actually learn what Runner's High means.

4. The end of the honeymoon

When you decide to train for a marathon, you get all excited, attend motivational kick-off events, buy cute clothes. You tell friends and family that you're training, and they get excited too. Your coaches are excited, as are your fellow runners. It's an exciting time. Then the actual training starts. And things get less exciting and increasingly more challenging. This is when some people lose interest in running and gain interest in their slippers.

As your new shoes turn from shiny white to dusty gray and you start to get annoyed with every song on your iPod, your initial enthusiasm will start to wane and you will wonder why you ever thought you had the energy to see this through to the end. This is a completely natural feeling and will fade once you remind yourself that you are in this for the long haul.

Throughout the training, you'll have times when you just don't feel like doing anything at all. You won't care what the training calendar says or how many times your running buddy calls. All you'll care about is that your recliner has been having abandonment issues and you need to reconnect with its lonely cushions. In these instances, you'll probably follow your instinct (it's primal really) and fall into your La-Z-Boy instead of getting out and pounding the pavement. This isn't the end of the world. Sure, you'll feel guilty about going off the training schedule even for a day and convince yourself that your training is ruined as a result. It is not. Just finish your Lifetime movie marathon and eat the last piece of kung pao chicken from the Chinese food takeout carton. Then grab the training schedule. Tomorrow is always another day, even if today is always reminding you how comfortable nonmovement is.

If you only miss a day or two, it's okay to rejoin the training that's in progress. You won't need to make up days, unless you missed a long run. The steadily increasing long runs are important, because they steadily increase your ability to endure pain for longer and longer periods of time. Some call this "psychological warfare"; others call it "training for a marathon." Either way, warfare doesn't have anything on what it feels like to skip a long run and "just catch the next one"—unless you are referring to the ambulance you're going to catch.

5. Pain

Over the course of several months, you're going to run hundreds of miles. Guess what? Sometimes you'll be sore. Well, let's be honest, *most* of the time you'll be sore. This is a fact. You will be challenging muscles that have been dormant for decades, and they will not be awakened without a fight. At times you'll experiment with ways to not breathe, to limit the movement of your sore stomach muscles. You'll ice your extremely sore calves and shins (ice is your best friend for these months). But pain is not a reason to abandon your training. If anything, it's a reason to keep going, because going through that much pain and not even finishing the damn training seems like a waste of Advil, not to mention being extremely anticlimactic.

●●●

Journal Entry: WEEK 6
Not My Best Week

I have been terribly busy this week—work, school, volunteering, time with friends and family, naps. Oh, did I mention all the running I've done this week? No, I didn't. The reason I omitted it is because I didn't run this week. Now don't get worried; don't get excited; don't think I'm quitting. I'm not. I just needed a little rest. I'm not Superwoman for god's sake. I'm barely even pulling off Homer Simpson right now.

I'm not sure why I didn't run this week. Well, I'm sure it has something to do with the fact that running is about as much fun as putting my head in a blender. Actually, running may be worse than that, because at least a blender would put me out of my misery a lot quicker. I ran seven miles on Saturday and decided that that was enough of that for the weekend. So I took Sunday off. Because I think even God took Sunday off when he was training for a marathon. Or something like that. I think that's in the Bible somewhere. Then Monday, well, I don't remember why I didn't run on Monday, but I'm sure it involved me being injured or possibly being sick. Yes, I think I broke my leg and had the flu on Monday. Bad day. Then there was Tuesday. I was supposed to run with Chipper Jen on Tuesday; we even set a time. But, a friend who was leaving for Iraq the next day (or maybe it was Long Beach; it was someplace with sand) invited me to dinner. *Hmmm, chase Jen around in circles or eat Mexican food?* It was a tremendously difficult decision, let me tell you. I mean, I had to choose between tacos and tostadas and burritos and those little taquito things. . . .

>>>

>>>

Then came Wednesday. I think my broken leg was acting up again that day. And Thursday was no good because a coworker has never been to Leatherby's Ice Cream Shoppe, the world-famous ice cream parlor here in town. And being the selfless person I am, I offered to take her to this wonderful place. The marathon and stroke survivors would just have to wait. This woman needed to experience a Leatherby's banana split. And then Friday. Who wants to run on Friday after such a long, hard week? I know you understand. The best part about not running this week is that my knees still hurt like hell. That's comforting. I'm going to be one of those old people with hearing aids who can tell the weather by the way her knees feel. Only I won't be old, I'll be twenty-nine. It will be great. It will be next week.

I debated whether to be honest in this journal entry, because I don't want my donors to get worried that their donations were for a woman who takes naps instead of running around in circles. Don't you fear; I'll be running again next week. Chipper Jen will make sure of that. If it comes down to it, she'll just come over to my house and talk at increasingly higher speeds until I'm eventually forced to put on my headphones and run away from her. And don't worry, she could keep that up for an entire marathon. She's that talented.

I would now like to add a little optimism, as I don't think my bright, shiny side gets enough airtime. I've finally found something wonderful about training for a marathon (besides the spandex, of course). I can eat whatever I want, whenever I want, and not gain a pound. This is by far the best part of all this running (besides the rash that the spandex gives me, of course). If you would like to gain some perspective on

>>>

>>>

how much I'm eating I'll give you a little math equation to help you calculate. I've run eighty-five miles in six weeks . . . well, about five weeks really, because, as I mentioned earlier, not many of those miles fell during this week. Eight-five miles. That's eighty-five more miles than I've run *total* in the last decade. So I've gone from sitting on my couch to running eighty-five miles. Man, I must be just shedding pounds by the minute, right? The other day I weighed myself and I had lost not one pound. Not one. I might be eating a little more than normal. The unfortunate part of this equation is what is going to happen to my butt around, oh, March, when I'm still eating, but I've reclaimed my position on my recliner. It could get real ugly, real quick.

For our seven-mile run on Saturday, Chipper Jen and I were able to combine my love of fatty foods and her love of running briskly while smiling. We did a race sponsored by Chevys Fresh Mex, which, coincidently, ran from one Chevys to another. I can't tell you how excited I was. Well, excited may be the wrong word. But I wasn't dreading it the way I do most runs. Why? Because this run had Chevys chips and salsa at the end! And a sombrero! Come on, that's exciting stuff. I'm telling you right now if they put fatty foods at the end of all my races I'd be a much more enthused runner.

As we started the race with many other chips and salsa enthusiasts, Chipper Jen promised she would not leave me on this run. "No I'll totally run with you this time. I want to run with you, I don't want to run ahead of you, let's just run . . ." I didn't catch the end of that sentence because at that point she had sprinted off to join the other ten-minute milers.

>>>

>>>

She waited for me at the finish line, though. And waited. And waited. And then waited some more. You see, I thought the race was only seven miles, when in fact it was a 12 K. A 12 K is like 7.3 miles or something pointless like that. Who measures anything in K's? Who even knows how far a K is? How is it that the running world is the only sport to not get the memo that we use miles as units of measurement?

Anyway, I stopped running at the seven-mile marker because that's how far I was set to run that day. I wondered why there wasn't anything set up, like a finish line or a salsa bar. But I didn't really mind, I just kept walking. Then I saw the balloons and the big sign that read FINISH. Chipper Jen was standing underneath the sign waving me in. "Run, run, you're almost finished." I gave her the I-don't-know-what-you're-talking-about look and pointed behind me, "I finished back there—at the seven-mile marker."

After the run I made my way to the food tent, where a tragedy had just taken place. They'd run out of chips and salsa. I took so long to finish the run that Chevys actually ran out of chips and salsa. I didn't know that was even possible. That's like Starbucks running out of coffee or me running at 7 AM—it's just not supposed to happen. But I did get a sombrero and some beans. What more do you need after running seven miles, really?

REAL LIMITS

1. Pain (again)

Although most of the time pain is just par for running the course, sometimes it is also your body's way of saying, "Whoa there bucko, if you're planning on using this body at all after this whole marathon madness, then we're going to need to slow it down a little bit." Severe pain should always be taken seriously and not merely written off as your bad karma for thinking you had any running ability whatsoever.

In Chapter 8 ("The Pain"), I go into greater detail about your marathon training pain and how to avoid it. If you're training with a team and have a coach, do not hesitate to ask whether your pain is simply the result of your body rediscovering movement or a greater problem. I know, it's difficult to imagine a problem greater than your body being forced to move, but do not ignore anything that seems like more than just soreness and general dissatisfaction with an active lifestyle.

2. Your body very loudly proclaiming it is time to take a break

I'm all for power of the mind, mind over matter, and all the other *Karate Kid*–type motivational techniques. But sometimes, no matter how hard your mind tries, it cannot get beyond your malfunctioning body. It's important to listen to your body when it's telling you it needs a break. Though it can be hard to distinguish between your body *wanting* and *needing* a break, usually the *wanting* has a way of fading once you make it clear that you will not be stopping. However, the *need* for a break has a way of getting more obvious as your body seems less and less able to continue running.

Yes, there are various walls that you will need to run through, and yes, those walls will feel insurmountable until you break through them. But sometimes the wall actually *is* insurmountable, and your body requires a little refueling before it can take it on again. If you ever doubt whether it's safe to keep running, err on the side of caution. Slow down and walk for a while, maybe stop and take some deep breaths while resting on a bench. (What a shocker, me recommending quality bench-resting time.)

KNOW YOUR LIMITS

I could write for days on end about various limits you may encounter while training (believe me, this is one thing I have plenty of reference material on). But the fact is, you are the only one who can differentiate between your imaginary and real limits. You'll figure them out as you move along and get to know your body's reaction to the training. Every person's body is going to be capable of different things, so don't ever use someone else's limits and abilities to define your own. Listen to your body and make choices based on what it's telling you (especially when it tells you it needs a full-body massage).

Remember that your goal is to complete a marathon, which means you have to actually get to the marathon, which means you should probably try not to burn out in Week 2 because you're determined to prove that you are limitless. You know your body well enough to know the difference between pushing yourself and killing yourself, so do your best to walk that line between the two. Doing so will help you exceed the limits that seem so overwhelming at the beginning of training.

Journal Entry: WEEK 10
Sixteen Miles of Good Times

This whole running thing is not going well, *at all*. How this can be healthy, I just do not know.

This weekend my little calendar o' runnin' said that I had to run sixteen miles. Is it me or is this number just getting ridiculous? Sixteen miles. What possible reason would one ever have for running sixteen miles? There simply is no reason. After about Mile 10, just call a cab and save yourself a lot of effort. Hell, call me. I'll give you a lift. Believe me, it's just not worth it. One fun fact about sixteen miles—that's about how far away hell is. I know, you'd think it'd be farther away, at least as far as Fresno. But you'd be wrong. Actually, I think I hit hell at about Mile 14, so it's an even shorter trip.

My route to hell began Saturday morning at 8:30 AM. It should have started at 7 AM, but Chipper Jen was off on a cruise ship heading toward Mexico while drinking many margaritas. And if she gets all-you-can-eat buffets and cabana boys, I get at least an extra hour of sleep on Saturday. I think that's fair. So I got up and prepared myself for a nice little morning jog that would most likely last until midafternoon. I'd eaten quite a bit of pasta late Friday night, because that seemed to help me during my half-marathon. Of course, the half-marathon started at 7 AM, and I wasn't starting this run until 8:30. That hour and a half shouldn't make much difference, right? This would be my first of several errors in judgment.

My next error came when I decided to only eat about half a PowerBar for breakfast. I tried to eat

>>>

>>>

the whole thing, but seriously, those things taste like someone took the shreddings from the bottom of a hamster cage, made them into a little brick, then covered them with fake chocolate. They aren't quite a Denny's "$1.99: Are you out of your mind?" breakfast. The PowerBar slogan should just be "Are you out of your mind?"

So with ten-hour-old pasta and a half a PowerBar filling my stomach I headed off for sixteen miles of running. I was running a bike trail along the river so I could run eight miles out and eight miles back on the same route. The first eight miles I didn't have any major problems. I was running behind a woman who was so old I feared the skin on her legs might wobble off. Please note: I was running *behind* this woman. Because I couldn't run fast enough to *get in front* of this woman. I eventually passed her around Mile 6. Note: This is because *she stopped running.* Whatever.

Miles 7, 8, 9, and 10 were in the direct sunlight, so that wasn't that much fun at all. And since I'd started late, it was starting to get warm. I run with a little Gatorade bottle that sits in a fanny pack–type thing. I try to drink my Gatorade sparingly in my first half of running, just a sip here and a sip there, because I know I'm gonna really need it as I get closer and closer to death . . . I mean to the end of the run.

I was also stopping to drink/bathe in the drinking fountains along the trail. You have to be pretty thirsty to actually drink from these fountains; I'm pretty sure they are in violation of at least forty-seven health codes. And I'm pretty sure Erin Brockovich could file about twelve lawsuits based on the quality of water coming out of those faucets. But at that point, I wouldn't have cared if the water was being pumped

>>>

>>>

through the aforementioned hamster cage. I was sweating about three gallons of fluids per minute, and I needed something, anything, to drink.

I also put my hat under the water and washed my face in an effort to keep my head cool and my face from becoming one big zit like it did after the half-marathon. After I put the hat back on and resumed running, the water dripping from my hat and face made for quite a dramatic sight. I looked like I'd been running so fast I was literally dripping sweat. How sweat could have gotten all the way up to the bill of my hat, I don't know. That's not important. The important part is that I looked very dramatic and very much like a *Runner's World* cover girl. This moment was shattered when the sweat/actually just water dripped onto my glasses, leaving me unable to see. This caused slight tripping and an awkward attempt to wipe my glasses with my shirt while running. Oh how quickly we athletes fall from glory.

Around Mile 10, all these good times began to come to an end. My body was not having nearly as much fun with this mile as it had with the previous nine. So far I had only stopped to bathe in the water fountains, so I thought I'd walk a little and try to regain my initial enthusiasm. When I was unable to get back to that happy place, I decided to open the little package of GU I had with me. You (and by "you" I mean *Runner's World* subscribers) just open it up, squeeze it in your mouth, and you are instantly hit with loads of energy and excitement for running. Or something. GU is on the taste meter somewhere between PowerBars and a taco. However, its consistency takes some getting used to. I washed it down with some water and started running again.

>>>

>>>

During Mile 11, I swallowed my first bug. Apparently it wasn't a very big bug, because it didn't give me any extra energy.

Miles 12 and 13 started to feel not so great. The mile markers for these two miles had very clearly been moved by someone, because I swear I'd run at least five miles in the time it took me to run those two miles. Every corner I came around I thought I saw the next mile marker, but no, it was just leaves. Mother Nature is so cruel.

Once I got past the Mile 13 marker, I started trying to psych myself up, *I can do this, three miles is nothing, I can do this.* Unfortunately, at this point my body said, *Uh, no, you can't do this, mostly because I will no longer be moving. Thank you for your support during this difficult time.* I kneeled down on the trail for a little rest, hoping to explain the situation to my body, *You can do this, you're just being a quitter, you're being a wimp. Come one, let's go.* To which my body answered, *Dude, I just ran thirteen friggin' miles, that's not wimpy!* I answered, *Good point, however, we are still three miles away from the car, with absolutely no options besides moving in order to get to that car.* This logic worked for about another half mile of movement, at which point my body said, *Yeah, I'm seriously done now. Thanks so much for playing. Enjoy your parting gifts and have a nice day. I'm taking a nap.*

It was awful, it was horrible, it was the hell I spoke of earlier. I wanted my mom. I wanted a bus. My mom driving a bus would have been perfect. I sat down on a bench, hugged my knees to my chest, and put my head down for a moment. Who knows how long that moment lasted, but when I woke up I felt much better. Yes, I

>>>

>>>

have actually incorporated napping into long-distance running. I think it's gonna catch on, I really do.

After my little nap I was ready to finish my last couple of miles. I decide to walk these miles, just in case my body wasn't fully back in working order. I power walked the last 2.5 miles. I timed my last 2.5 miles. I walk faster than I run. I really do. Whatever. I finished sixteen miles. That's still ten miles less than a marathon. Hopefully they have benches along the marathon route to accommodate my napping needs.

JOURNAL SPACE

Use the journal space here to note the limits you feel throughout your training. As you move through the weeks, I encourage you to reread your thoughts about the walls, which may eventually turn out to be just speed bumps, along the way. This will give you a little perspective on the new limits that present themselves and will give you the confidence to blaze right past them.

LIMIT #1: _____
_____
_____
_____
_____
_____
_____
_____
_____
_____

LIMIT #2 _____

_____

_____

_____

_____

_____

_____

_____

_____

_____

_____

_____

_____

LIMIT #3: _____

_____

_____

_____

_____

_____

_____

_____

_____

_____

_____

_____

_____

_____

CHAPTER *Six*
The Moment

There are like 500 songs with the word "moment" in the title. There's "One Moment in Time"—"I want one moment in time/When I'm more than I thought I could be." Whitney Houston famously belted this out to our Olympic athletes, inspiring them to grab a gold medal or she'd send Bobby Brown after them. A few years ago, Kelly Clarkson sang "A Moment Like This"—"Some people wait a lifetime/For a moment like this"— shortly after being crowned the first American Idol. Although Fox likes to stretch the show out, she really only had to wait one season, not a lifetime, for her moment like that. But my all-time favorite "moment" song is "This Is the Moment"—"When all I've done/All the dreaming,/Scheming and screaming,/Become one." Only my fellow theater dorks will recognize this song from the Broadway musical *Jekyll & Hyde*. It truly is one of the greatest "moment" songs: ever-powerful, moving, and inspirational. (Fellow theater dorks also know that the song becomes slightly less inspirational when you're aware that it's being sung by a schizophrenic mad scientist.)

Yet, I digress. My point is, there are lots of inspirational songs that can be played during the big moments of life. We've all heard these songs played over slow-motion video of people exuberantly celebrating the big love/game of their life/final round of *Supermarket Sweep,* and they start jumping/crying/

throwing high-priced cheese while the credits roll. And there we are at home, jumping/crying/throwing cheese right along with them. Because we can imagine what it must feel like to wait a lifetime for a moment like that. And somewhere deep inside, we genuinely hope that someday we'll have a high-priced cheese moment of our own.

Am I here to tell you that finishing a marathon is that high-priced cheese moment you've been waiting for? No. I'm here to warn you not to focus so much on the cheese that you lose your taste for the economically priced (and just as tasty) snack crackers along the way.

When you train for a marathon, you're constantly reminded of all the joy and exuberance you'll feel when you cross that final finish line. But if you're anything like me, you're going to need a lot more than potential joy to get you through months of very real pain and exhaustion. I'm all for fighting and earning and work-ing hard. But I'm not against a little instant gratification either. Why wait for your final sprint- (or slog-) across-the-finish-line moment to bust out your boombox and let Whitney wail? Yes, you'll have an overwhelming sense of accomplishment and pride after you complete your marathon, but it is also so so so important to acknowledge what you're accomplishing with every individual mile you finish along the way. Like everything in life, it's easy to allow the moments of your training to pass you by without really appreciating them.

More than just that one big moment, your marathon will be the culmination of little moments, subtle changes, and notewor-thy milestones. Sure, the point of all of these moments is to lead you to the finish line; but if you look a little deeper and get in

touch with your Oprah side, you'll find that training can be about
a lot more than just one race. Most of the things you'll learn about
yourself, your limits, and your abilities won't come during the actual marathon. They'll come during less-obvious times, times that
might be overlooked because you're focusing so intently on the
marathon itself. They'll come when you lace up and hit the trail,
even though the lacing up itself is enough to aggravate your poor
sore muscles. They will be the times you exuberantly proclaim,
"I only have to run nine miles this weekend!" when a few weeks
earlier the mere thought of a nine-mile run would have sent you
whimpering into the fetal position. They'll come at times when
you run through pouring rain, sideways wind, and scorching heat,
because you made a commitment and you intend to keep it, regardless of Mother Nature's rather mean-spirited sense of humor.

It's in these little moments when you'll realize, as many a
profound person has observed, that sometimes the journey is
worth more than the destination. The marathon-training journey
is about a lot more than merely finishing one (very long) race. It's
about getting to the race; it's about challenging yourself in ways
that seem obscene to any sane person; it's about coming up with
unique ways to treat various rashes caused by spandex.

So do yourself a favor: After you finish a long run, and before
you look at your training calendar to see what mileage lies ahead,
take a moment to bask in the glory of getting one step closer to
your overall goal. (That goal being, of course, not dying while
training for a marathon.) Realize that each run is a goal in itself,
so in essence you cross a goal off your list every time you kick off
those sweaty running shoes. Take a moment after each run to cool
down and acknowledge what your body has accomplished. Turn

off the headphones, be silent, and just listen to your heart pounding in your ears. Yes, it's slightly bizarre that your heart has taken up residency in your skull; apparently that's where it resides when you are a physically active person. Do not be alarmed.

I give you this advice because it's the advice I had trouble taking from others. One of my biggest problems during training was my inability to take in my accomplishments as they were happening. The second I finished running eleven miles, my only thought (besides, *Why didn't I park closer?*) was, *Next week I have to do thirteen miles.* It's hard to stay positive when such negative events loom on the horizon.

One day I had to run sixteen miles in the morning and attend a housewarming party in the afternoon. The sixteen-mile run had gone horribly; and by the time I dragged myself to the party, all I could do was plop into the nearest chair, where unfortunately the seven-layer bean dip was just out of reach. As I sat longing for the delicious combination of sour cream and beans, random people inquired about my training. (My immobility made my training the most obvious conversation topic.) Without fail, each of them said something along the lines of "Well, I think it's amazing what you are doing" or "I'm really impressed." Normally I would just shrug these compliments off with a "No, believe me, nothing about my running is amazing." But that day, as I sat there longing for bean dip and a warm bath, I actually allowed myself to start believing their compliments.

Maybe it *was* a little amazing that I'd finished sixteen miles. Maybe it was even more amazing considering the fact that the most strenuous activity I usually got credit for at parties was my ability to name all seven layers of bean dip without any hints. But the most amazing thing of all was that, considering how many calories I'd burned during my sixteen-mile run, I could probably eat the entire tray of seven-layer bean dip and not gain a pound. Cue Whitney. . . .

About that time, I started becoming a little more impressed with myself, and not only with what I was *attempting* to do, but with what I'd *already* done. This created a profound shift in my overall outlook and my ability to stay encouraged. It is very easy to become overwhelmed by your training calendar, but if you acknowledge all that you've accomplished in your previous weeks it will help you realize that you are completely capable of tackling what comes next. This is tremendously helpful when you're lying on a park bench wondering if you'll be able to breathe without a respirator, let alone finish your run.

So go my little runners! Go embrace the moments of your life! Run in slow motion (or if you're like me, just run), give people high-fives, and invite Whitney Houston (or the entire cast of *Jekyll & Hyde*) out to the running trail to sing your praises. Celebrate what you're accomplishing as you accomplish it. I promise it will make your training much more enjoyable (and frankly, Whitney could probably use the gig).

●●●

Journal Entry: WEEK 9
The Tin Man Running Style

Week 9 and I'm still alive. I have run 127 miles now, and I've still yet to get anywhere except back to my car. I've also started running on a treadmill, so I can both figuratively and literally run nowhere. Sometimes when I'm out clubbin' I even do the Running Man dance to continue my theme of moving a lot yet getting nowhere. (If you don't know the Running Man ask someone between the ages of twenty-three and thirty-three to demonstrate it. I warn you, though, the Running Man dance is similar to a marathon in that you really shouldn't attempt it without the proper training. I do not recommend it for the novice booty-shaker.)

I completed my first half-marathon last week. The highlight of this event was the fact that I actually completed it. There were also several lowlights. Let's discuss them, shall we? I know people think I'm kidding when I say that I'm the slowest runner in the history of the world. I'm not kidding. When the earth started flooding and Noah had to wade through five feet of water carrying two donkeys, two rhinos, and two hamsters to get to his ark, he was moving faster than I do. Hell, I think the two swimming snails were moving faster. It took me three friggin' hours to run/jog/crawl 13.1 miles. I'll save you the effort of doing the math on that one—I ran slow. Walkers were blazing past me. I kid you not: A sixty-five-year-old walking woman left me in the dust. But at least she gave me a thumbs-up as she passed me. That was special. Chipper Jen finished the half-marathon in two hours. A full hour before me. And I'm sure she was smiling the whole time. Whatever.

>>>

>>>

A friend of Jen's offered to videotape our half-marathon, giving me the opportunity to see what I look like while running. First of all, to classify what I'm doing as running would be like calling Paris Hilton a thespian. I always knew I had a unique running style. But until I saw it on video, I didn't fully understand how unique it is. Apparently my rebellious nature has spilled over into my marathoning because I absolutely refuse to pick up my legs while running. I don't need no stinking joints, so I'll just drag my legs for thirteen miles. I call it the Tin Man Running Style. I believe my running body also makes sounds similar to the Tin Man's squeaks, so it's really both a visual and audio treat.

I've recently altered my running style slightly. I was told I should run so that my heel hits the ground before my toe. I'd been running with my toes hitting first, in an attempt to bounce like Jen bounces. But that wasn't working because I'm not a real bouncy person on the whole. The heel-to-toe method is supposed to absorb some of the shock and allow my knees to stay on my body until at least December. I have yet to figure out a method of absorbing the shock of getting out of bed at 6:30 AM on a weekend, though. Any suggestions for remedying that jarring effect would be greatly appreciated.

The good news is that this heel-to-toe method has really helped my poor knees. The bad news is I look like a complete moron. The combination of Tin Man and heel-to-toe running styles provides a visual best described as Dawn-Trying-to-Catch-Up-With-Her-Own-Feet Running Style. I think it could catch on; it really is one of the more attractive things you'll ever see. Look for me on the cover of next month's *Runner's World,* 'cause I'm a sight to behold.

>>>

>>>

Speaking of *Runner's World*, my boss gave me an old issue. It is chock-full of interesting and surprising tidbits, the most interesting and surprising of which is the fact that there is such a magazine. Who knew? A whole 104 pages about running. Well, fifty pages are about running; the rest are advertisements featuring people running, jogging, lunging, sweating, or just sitting around looking extremely well toned while eating a vitamin-enriched snack. The cover model for this issue is some crazy lady named Paula who finished a marathon in two hours and fifteen minutes. What the? I'm lucky to finish stretching in two hours and fifteen minutes. Paula has this to say about marathons: "In a marathon I feel a lot more in control of the race than I do in shorter races. I feel totally at home with the marathon." Paula's home and my home are in two completely different neighborhoods.

As I read through the magazine I came across a pie graph displaying the results of a reader poll. The readers were asked, "What's the longest race you've ever run?" Keep in mind that the participants in this poll are people who love running so much that they actually want to read a magazine dedicated solely to running/runners/sweating. They love running, they can't get enough of it. You get my point. So what percentage of these run-happy people have run a marathon? Eighty percent? Ninety percent? Oh no, try 32 percent. 32 friggin' percent. Of crazy, happy runners. Of people who can't get enough running. Only 32 percent of them have ever run a marathon. Again, I will save you the effort of doing the math—I'm screwed.

The half-marathon I ran was also a full marathon for people (*Runner's World* subscribers, no doubt) who couldn't imagine stopping at thirteen miles when they had the opportunity to run twenty-six. These are not

>>>

>>>

normal people. These are Serious Runners. If I missed seeing the Serious Runners at the beginning of the race, it was okay, 'cause I'd see them again three more times throughout my thirteen miles. *How is that possible?* you may ask. Well you see, the route was 6.5 miles out, and then 6.5 miles back along the same road. To run twenty-six miles, the Serious Runners had to run the thirteen-mile course twice. This meant that they passed me once on the way out, then once as they made their way back. In the time it took them to run 6.5 miles out and three miles back, I had only gone about five miles out. Splendid. Then they passed me again as they went back out and again as they came back in. Yes, when I was dragging my slow butt across the nine-mile marker, the Serious Runners were passing me (on their twenty-second mile). I made up a song about this. Well, I didn't make it up, Lionel Richie made it up, I just changed his words a little. It goes like this: "Once . . . Twice . . . Three tiiiimes you've passed meee . . . and I wanna triiiiiip yoooouuu."

Feel free to sing along. Hell, if you're so inspired you can do the Running Man dance while singing my new pop hit. But don't worry, you still won't look as stupid as I do wearing spandex while trying to catch up with my own feet.

FINDING YOUR MOMENTS

1. No matter how exhausted you are, try to muster the energy to say yes when your fellow runners invite you out for a meal or a coffee after a run. Yes, I know that the thought of remaining vertical for even one minute longer makes you physically ill; but no one understands what you're going through like the other people who are training with you. Spending some post–run time bonding

and bitching will invigorate you and provide you with the comfort of knowing you aren't the only one who thought about hailing a cab at Mile 9.

2. Find local running events and participate in as many as you can throughout your training. Sometimes, they may be the same distance you're supposed to run that weekend. They're also a fun place to meet other runners and really experience the cult that is running. You have no idea how many runners there are in your town until you go to a running event and see them come out of hiding and onto the course—a mass of spandex and enthusiasm for running in the AM hours. But more important, the organized runs give you an excellent way to celebrate your running accomplishments. There's nothing like live music and free food to help you feel good about finishing another run. In fact, if it's in your budget, I highly recommend getting the music and food at the end of all your runs. Sure, it may seem like overkill, but you are training for a major athletic event! A little showmanship never hurt anyone.

3. You know when there's a birthday or a holiday or a Wednesday at work and people bring in extremely unhealthy food to celebrate? Normally you probably shy away from eating too much, because your waistline can't handle cake, cookies, and doughnuts at regular intervals. But guess what? You're training for a marathon! Which means that in addition to your newfound joint aches and Advil-dependence, you are now burning calories at supersonic speeds! So hobble your medicated butt over to the party tray and go at it. This is the one time in life when you can eat to your heart's content and not feel even a twinge of guilt. But be sure to value this time, because once the marathon is over and your butt reattaches to the couch, your days of bathing in calories will be but a distant—though glorious—memory.

4. Write everything down. I know I've mentioned the journal before, and the existence of many a blank journal page at the back of this book is probably enough to make it clear that I encourage written reflection, but I can't say enough about journaling (or blogging) during the training process. While the journal will provide a great way to remember your training years down the line, it is also a great way to relive your moments as they are happening. Sometimes it is difficult to fully appreciate what you are accomplishing while you are actually doing the running. Sometimes it is difficult to do anything besides find the nearest water fountain while you're running. Survival instinct does not often include time for reflection and sentimental thoughts. That is why I encourage you to pick up a pen and a journal after you've collapsed on your bed, but just before you become completely unable to move any muscle in your body. Writing in a journal will force you to tell your story and to hear it yourself. And believe me, running is nothing if not a sport that is more enjoyable upon reflection than it is upon participation. So turn to the end of this book, and get started. Here, I'll give you a starting point: "Moment #1: Today I read a really inspiring and brilliant chapter of a book about running. It changed my life." You wouldn't want that memory to slip away.

5. Buy at least one new pair of pants that highlights your newly toned butt. Don't spend a lot of money on them, but make sure they're cute, and make sure you know how cute you are in them. Wear them with pride while showing off the fruits of your insane labor. Then go eat an entire pizza and don't even worry about the zipper bursting. Sing it with me ladies, "Some people wait a lifetime/For a moment like this. . . ."

Journal Entry: WEEK 14
Let Us Give Thanks

Thanksgiving is coming up, and I thought to myself, *Self, you really don't look at the positive side of running enough. You aren't thankful for all the things that come along with running 250 miles in three and a half months.* So in spirit of the holiday, I have decided to list the running things I'm thankful for. I mean, the Indians came together with the Pilgrims and gave thanks, even though the Pilgrims were planning to kill the Indians shortly after the pumpkin pie was served. If they could put aside that minor detail, then I can put aside my immense dislike for running and give thanks for its place in my life these past few months. So here we go . . .

RUNNING-RELATED THINGS I AM THANKFUL FOR

1. The number-one thing I'm thankful for is the fact that after this weekend I do not have to do any more long runs. To clarify, long runs are runs of distances so long you really should take a plane, train, or automobile. This weekend was the last of our stupidly long runs. And now we are tapering so as to rest our completely ruined bodies before we make them run a whole marathon. *Well, since it was your last long run, did you run the twenty-six miles you are gonna have to run in Hawaii?* you may ask, because that would be a perfectly logical question and assumption. *Oh no,* I would answer.

   It seems that the training program only takes you to about twenty miles, six miles short of the twenty-six you'll run on race day. Apparently we

>>>

>>>

do not train to twenty-six because "the excitement of race day will carry you through the last six miles." What the? Excitement of race day? Carrying me through six friggin' miles? I just tried to think of something witty and funny that would actually excite me enough to run six miles. I came up with nothing. At all.

And since when do you only train for two-thirds of an athletic event?

"Johnny here is going for the Olympic Gold Medal in the triple jump. Tell me about your training program, Johnny."

"Well, Jim, basically we just trained for the first two jumps, and I'm hoping that the excitement of the Olympics pretty much carries me through the last jump."

"Oh, that would explain why all of those high jumpers over there are only jumping moderately high, and those divers are all belly flopping because they are only practicing two-thirds of their dives."

"Yes, Jim, they're on the same training schedule I am."

2. Because my long runs are over, I'm thankful I'll never have to go to my running trail again. Not that my running trail and I haven't had some good times. I mean, I never died while running on it, a fact which in itself far exceeds all my expectations for the trail. But it's time for the two of us to part, my running trail and I. I've logged many a mile on its course, and I've cussed many a word.

>>>

>>>

Now that my long runs are over, I don't need the miles and miles the trail offers. As I ran my last long run, I was aware that this would be the last time I visited this trail I'd come to know so well. I got a little nostalgic. Between my napping on the benches and peeing in the bushes, I've been served well by the trail. I will even overlook the occasional malfunctioning of its water fountains because the abundance of unleashed dogs on the trail always provided the same spurt of energy that a refreshing gulp of water might have allowed.

Although this is the end of the road for me and the running trail, I know that it is not goodbye. I know that every time I think of running, or even dream of running, I will revisit the trail in my mind. Even now, so far removed from its endless asphalt course, I can still picture its every curve, mile marker, water fountain, and bathroom. Sure, I had a tendency to threaten terrorist acts against the never-ending miles that were forced on me; sure, sometimes it seemed as though the strategically placed piles of horse poop and near-fatal run-ins with speeding bikers were the trail's passive-aggressive way of keeping me in check. But, although our relationship was a volatile one, it was also quite a productive one. So I said goodbye to my trusty trail with gratitude and one extended finger, a fitting end to our time together.

3. I am thankful for my sports bra. And we'll just leave it at that.

4. I am thankful that Jen has once again become chipper. Last week I was alarmed when she entered a dark place and uttered the words, "I hate

>>>

>>>

running," having just returned from a two-week cruise on which she had engaged in many a buffet and alcoholic beverage, and not one running activity. This made her acclimation back to the running world a bit harsh, and in her time of struggle she actually uttered the words, "I hate running." Can you imagine? Our little Chipper One, bearer of positive attitude and light? A collective gasp could be heard across the land as the world contemplated an unchipper, unbouncy Jen.

But everyone can relax. Our Jen is back in tip-top bouncing shape and has managed to pull herself out of the darkness. As evidence, here's the message she left me the other day after running twenty-one miles: "hithisisjeni justgotdonerunningtwentyonemilesitwasawesome ilovedititwasthebestandi'mdoneandididitandiloved itand I LOVE ENDORPHINS!!!!!!" Please note that she said all this on voice mail, not to my face. Because she knows that chipperness of that magnitude cannot be within striking distance of me. So, I'm thankful I didn't have to strike my friend in order to stop her chipperness. I merely had to hang up my phone. Energy efficient and quite effective.

5. Lastly, I am thankful for the amount of pie I get to eat on Thanksgiving and not gain a pound. God bless us everyone.

CHAPTER *Seven*
The Lifestyle

One does not go from recliner to race day by merely picking up a training schedule and deciding to run a couple miles every week. If you do the training correctly, it will dramatically change your entire lifestyle. Think of it as *Extreme Makeover: Your Nice Quiet Life Edition*. Just like reality TV, things will probably get a little messy before the end.

When I was training, my friends and family were amazed by the changes they saw in my lifestyle. They often commented that I was becoming a whole new person. Then I would go off on a profanity-laced monologue about my last long run, and they'd realize that my bitter sarcasm had miraculously survived the transformation.

But I had to make those changes or I wouldn't have been able to complete the marathon. Don't think I didn't try my hardest to cling to my old lifestyle, hoping like hell I could figure out a way to finish a marathon without having to veer too far from my La-Z-Boy. But I eventually realized that the only thing my recliner could add to my training efforts was an excellent way to elevate my poor knees while I iced them.

Remember that you've spent a lifetime establishing your pre-training lifestyle, and changes you make aren't going to happen overnight; and they aren't going to happen without some real effort on your part to break out of old habits. Keep in mind that

the new habits you're forcing on yourself aren't just a good idea—
they are habits that will literally make or break your entire training. And if you're going to bother to venture off your recliner,
you may well bother to do it right. Below I've listed a few lifestyle
changes to expect while training.

THE DAY

Your overall daily routine will undergo a dramatic change.
Perhaps your pre-training routine involves getting up, going to
work, coming home, watching TV, and going to bed. Perhaps you
throw in a trip to the video store or hanging out with friends if
you're feeling adventurous. Once you start training, your routine
will have to stretch to accommodate running, cross-training,
icing, medicating, and so on. If you look at the schedules on
pages 6–13, you'll see that only two days a week are Rest Days,
while the other days have running or cross-training scheduled.
With the exception of long runs, daily trainings usually don't
take more than an hour to complete. But how many of us sit
around pre-training thinking, *Man, do I just have* too *many hours
in the day. I sure wish I could find some more things to do, because I
often feel like my days just aren't full enough.* No one thinks like
that (and if you do, you obviously need to order more cable stations). We all have lives that often involve us collapsing into bed
at night while mentally making a list of all the crap we didn't
get to during the day.

When you decide to fit marathon training into your already-
busy day, you'll have to get creative about finding the time to
do it. Don't worry, you'll figure it out. Because you are woman!
Hear you schedule! Some people wake up early and tackle their

mileage before their normal day starts; others go for runs on their lunch break, then eat lunch at their desks later. I didn't follow either option: Getting up early violated my strong anti-morning beliefs; and showering in the company locker room didn't seem like a good midday activity. I ran at night, either right after work when it was still light or well after sunset when only crackheads and anti-morning people are out at the track.

You'll figure out a daily schedule that's in sync with your routine, energy level, and self-discipline. If you can jump out of bed and greet the morning with a jog and a smile, then by all means jog and smile. Once you've found a way to fit a jog and a smile into any part of your day, you're going to want to make it your Regularly Scheduled Time of Movement. This way the running will slowly become part of your regular routine and eventually you'll wonder what you used to do with all the time you now spend running. (For the answer, look in the direction of your poor neglected recliner and remote control.)

THE FOOD

By far the best part of marathon training is food, food, food. Eat, eat, eat. During training, you can eat whatever you want whenever you want and you won't gain weight. Now, if you actually eat, eat, eat, like I did, you'll notice that you've managed to run hundreds of miles and have not lost even a single pound. It's a bit discouraging. But who cares about weight loss when you can eat a banana split at 2 AM without a bit of hesitation? That might be the source of the *real* Runner's High everyone talks about.

Another great thing about the eating? It's an important part of training. You *have* to take in a lot of calories. Isn't that awesome?

I was only going to eat a small salad for lunch but I really need more calories. So I guess I'll have the steak and potatoes. I have to. You'll go from burning roughly one calorie a day to burning a billion; therefore you need to make sure your food intake reflects that massive change in activity.

Unfortunately, all the eating does have a purpose other than merely taking in mass quantities of calories. (You knew it was too good to be true.) Food provides your body with the things it needs to not keel over when you're pushing it beyond any physical limits it has ever endured. As we discussed in Chapter 4, it's important when you train for a marathon to maintain a diet high in carbs, moderate in protein, and low in fatty foods. Yes, I know that a low-fat diet is hardly exciting. But look! Carbs! You *have* to eat carbs! All through your training, bread is once again safe! I know that carbs have been demonized in recent years, made to look like they are single-handedly responsible for the obesity levels of Americans, but in the world of marathon training, the carb has near biblical status. When runners say things like "carbo load," they're giving you advice, not calling you names.

To be successful in your training, you have to change your eating habits so that they're appropriate for an active person instead of someone who merely eats during TV commercial breaks. I know the grocery store can be a scary place, but you'll have to make it a regular destination during your training. Plan three complete meals a day, as well as occasional snacks. And then stick to your plan. Do not skip meals or you'll feel like a melting snowman when you try to muster up energy to finish your run. And with your lack of functioning legs and abundance of sweat you may actually look like a melting snowman, too.

Journal Entry: WEEK 4
Better?

Today someone asked me the same question I'm often asked: "Do you feel better?" I gave her my standard answer, "Than what?" Than a three-legged dog that just stepped on a tack? I feel slightly better than that. "No," she said, "do you feel better than you did before you started?" I gave her the blankest stare ever known to mankind. *Better than when I started?!*

When I started, I still had full use of all my body. When I stood up, my knees, back, and thighs didn't scream at me. My pee had not yet turned fluorescent from the vitamins I hadn't started taking. My breasts had not all but bounced right off my body. I was not yet eating things like PowerBars, which I'm pretty sure look and taste the same on the way into your body as they do on the way out. I wasn't peeing every 4.5 seconds because of the amount of fluids I was drinking. And, most important, Jen wasn't nearly as chipper as she is now. Well, maybe she was. But that's not the point.

The point is that my fitness routine a month ago consisted entirely of me getting to the bottom of my stairs at home and then realizing I had forgotten something upstairs. I would then have to bitterly climb back up the stairs to retrieve said object. And about 50 percent of the time I'd just leave the object upstairs, because who really has the energy to climb stairs? Now I have a slightly different routine, which involves me leaving the object upstairs 100 percent of the time. I've gone out to dinner with no purse, no glasses, and one shoe. It's just too much to climb those stairs.

Even if you aren't up for regularly preparing meals, try to limit your dependence on fast food. If you're physically incapable of turning on an oven or stove and simply must eat, at least try to be conscious of the food you eat and make sure it sorta resembles something an active person might consume. (Hint: If french fries make up more than half of the meal, it ain't exactly going to be featured in the diet section of *Runner's World* magazine.)

In addition to a training-friendly diet, I highly recommend engaging in an "I so deserve this" reward meal once in a while. Sure, that banana split at 2 AM won't increase your running performance with its nutrients and vitamins, but it may increase your performance at Mile 11 when you need to promise yourself a reward for finishing your run instead of hitchhiking to the end. Few times in our lives do we get to eat anything we want without feeling guilty. These training months are one of those times. (The only other time being when you're pregnant; "The *baby needs* this cannoli!") Eat a balanced diet, but also explore the bliss of eating your favorite ridiculously caloried food of choice.

FIVE MEALS NOT RECOMMENDED BY ANY TRAINER (BUT HIGHLY RECOMMENDED BY ME)

o BOBOLI PIZZA: Bread, tomato sauce, and cheese. Throw some pepperoni on top and you've got all the food groups. Seems like a health jackpot to me.

o CHEF BOYARDEE BEEFARONI: I still fail to see what is wrong with this excellent meal choice. Beef = Protein; Roni (as in Maca) = Pasta. Am I missing something? Isn't this the perfect training food?

o BAG O' SALAD: Everything—dressing, croutons, shredded lettuce—comes in the little bag! Is this not exciting? Sure, the dressing probably has more fat than a Big Mac, but look, lettuce! That's gotta be healthy, right?

o TACO LOCO BURRITO: It's got beans, meat, cheese, sour cream, guacamole, and salsa. It's a party in a tortilla if you ask me. And you *should* ask me, because I ate 382 of these throughout my training. Taco Loco is a great place to go post-run and pre-not-being-able-to-move-for-three-days.

o CHICKEN CACCIATORE: Please take note, this is the only meal I know how to make. Chicken. In an oven-safe bowl (side note: plastic is not oven-safe), pour stewed tomatoes over the top of chicken. Cook at, like, 350 degrees for as long is it takes to cook chicken (until it ain't pink). Then make Minute Rice, and eat it all together. It looks and tastes just like a real meal. Throw in a salad and call yourself domesticated.

THE ENERGY

For some scientific reason unknown to me, I actually felt more energized once I started training. It made no sense, considering I was exerting more energy in a twenty-minute run than I used to expend in an entire week. Mathematically this is confusing. But I will never admit that my training actually led to positive things like motivation and ambition. That would ruin my street cred as a disgruntled runner.

Training turns your lifestyle upside down and is a tremendous undertaking. But your energy level increases to meet your body's need. Instead of feeling exhausted after a run, you'll often feel recharged. There is some very scientific, biological reason for this that involves endorphins and blood flow and possibly a nutrient or two, but the only thing you really need to know is that your body is energized and you should take advantage of this moment in time. Apply this newfound vigor to the rest of your life: Empty your in-box at work, play that extra game of UNO with the kids, grab the broom and sweep the cobwebs that have been on your ceiling for six months (don't judge, we all have our ways of excelling).

If you approach your lifestyle change in a realistic, steady manner, you should be able to make it through training without experiencing the jarring effects that can result from a dramatic 180-degree change. Remember that just like any change in life, your months of training won't always go smoothly. You'll go through periods when you revert back to your old routines, when you aren't feeling like a woman who can whisper, much less roar. This is okay. Whisper (hell, even whimper) if you need to, then get back on track as soon as you can. The longer you veer away from your newfound run-happy life, the more difficult it will be to regain your enthusiasm for movement. When you're low on motivation, you can always conjure up images of the guilt-free banana split—that ought to get the enthusiasm levels rising once again.

MY LIFE BEFORE AND AFTER I STARTED TRAINING FOR A MARATHON

Oh what a difference a couple hundred miles makes. . . . Read on.

Typical liquid intake
BEFORE:
A Mountain Dew in the morning, a Coke for lunch, and maybe a sip of water after dessert at night.

AFTER:
A yogurt fruit smoothy concoction containing approximately four million calories with breakfast, followed by roughly thirty-two gallons of water throughout the day.

Bathroom breaks
BEFORE:
Maybe one a day.

AFTER:
Similar to the number taken by an eight-and-a-half-month pregnant woman (i.e., every thirteen minutes). Only I don't have a child sitting on my bladder, I just have a bladder unable to keep up with the rigors of my newfound devotion to drinking the daily recommended intake of water.

Vitamin intake
BEFORE:
Do the rainbow of fruit flavors in Skittles count?

AFTER:
Pills the size of marshmallows washed down with one of my thirty-two gallons of water.

Color of urine

BEFORE:

The color it's supposed to be.

AFTER:

Neon green.

Typical meal

BEFORE:

A rotation of fast food, takeout, and french fries, with the occasional milk shake thrown in to cover the dairy food group.

AFTER:

A ridiculous mix of identifiable food that has not been cooked using a deep fryer of any sort. Salad, chicken, pasta, and other mysterious foods have made their way into my once-barren refrigerator.

Calories burned in a day

BEFORE:

Probably like four.

AFTER:

Roughly 13,297.

Energy level

BEFORE:

That of a comatose snail.

AFTER:

Skyrocketed energy level, consistent with that of a snail on crack.

The gym

BEFORE:

A place entered once only to sign papers that would then allow the gym to deduct money from my bank account on a monthly basis.

AFTER:

Interestingly, a place where people are allowed to exercise because of the money taken out of their bank accounts every month. A place where I've actually *waited in a line* for the privilege of *running in place* for thirty minutes.

Saturdays

BEFORE:

A day of rest, which, much like Jesus, I needed. I bet Jesus didn't get up before noon on his day of rest, either. He seemed like a sensible guy.

AFTER:

A day of pain. And no rest. Unless you count naps taken on park benches. The days on which my long runs are scheduled, runs that mock me with their stubbornly increasing distances and their need to start before noon. Every week they wait for me, these long runs, and I can see them in the distance throughout the week as I begrudgingly make my way closer to the dreaded Saturday.

My ab muscles

BEFORE:

There are muscles there?

AFTER:

Friggin' fantastic.

YOUR BEFORE, AND, AFTER CHART

In the blank spaces on the following page, jot down places where you start to notice changes in your routine. Return to these notes during your marathon training to see the differences in your life before and after you began training. This exercise will demonstrate how much you can alter your lifestyle if you put your mind to it. It will also remind you of how great you had it before you lost your mind and decided to abandon your poor recliner.

BEFORE: _____

AFTER: _____

BEFORE: _____

AFTER: _____

BEFORE: _____

AFTER: _____

BEFORE: _____

AFTER: _____

BEFORE: _____

AFTER: _____

BEFORE: _____

AFTER: _____

BEFORE: _____

AFTER: _____

BEFORE: _____

AFTER: _____

BEFORE: _____

AFTER: _____

BEFORE: _____

AFTER: _____

Journal Entry: WEEK 8
This "Gym" Place

I've been way too busy this last week. You see, the new TV season started, leaving no time for silly things like journal entries and marathon training and work. It's important to have priorities. I know you understand.

Fall not only ushers in a new TV season, it also brings shorter days, which doesn't help someone who's trying to fit in work, school, running, and napping all before sundown. Luckily, I can sometimes combine the napping with work and school. But it still leaves little time to run before it gets dark. And if I run in the dark, I'll be attacked by attackers, or worse yet, those pesky Mormons handing out Bibles.

As much as I'd love to use the darkness as an excuse for not running, it turns out that people actually do exercise after sundown. There are these new places where you can exercise whenever you feel like it. They are called gyms. I'm pretty sure I've belonged to one or two in the past. Although I could go whenever I felt like it, I never really felt like it. To be honest, I'm still not that enthused. But I'm even less enthused about keeling over while attempting to run 26.2 miles, so exercise I must.

I didn't want to go to the gym alone, so I called my friend Jodi and asked her to go with me. As soon as she recovered from shock, she agreed to go with me. It seemed that in the fifteen years we've been friends I've never asked her to do anything physical, let alone go to a gym, a Mecca of movement. I beg to differ with her version of the facts. I distinctly remember signing the two of us up for a three-legged race in the fifth

>>>

grade. But now that I think about it, I also remember falling down on our first conjoined step and being pulled the rest of the way. That might have marked the end of our physical activity together.

Be that as it may, I was signing up for a gym. I was going to go buff up, work out, and sweat to the oldies. Or something like that. As soon as I walked in, a buff guy with a shaved head pounced on me and started spewing pointless gym facts like the number of blah-blah machines they have and such and such amenities they offer. "Whatever . . . do you have a treadmill?" "Yes we do." "Can I sign up for just three months?" "Well, what are you going to do after three months?" "Take a nap and eat some Cheetos." He looked at me like he didn't even know what Cheetos were. At this point, Jodi was starting to reevaluate whether fifteen-plus years of friendship was really that special. I'm lucky she's not very strong, or she most likely would have picked up a barbell and dropped it on my head.

The buff, bald guy said that I could get a discount on my monthly fee if I agreed to only come to the gym on Mondays, Wednesdays, Fridays, and Sundays. This sounded great to me. That meant that on Tuesdays, Thursdays and Saturdays I *couldn't* go to the gym. "Wanna go to the gym?" "You know, I really, really do. But I can't, I'm not allowed to go today. A shame, really." So I signed up for Mondays and Wednesdays, 'cause who really thinks I'm going to the gym on Fridays and Sundays? Let's be realistic.

Unfortunately, I signed up for my membership on a Monday evening, so I was able to stay and work out that very night. Although the registration process seemed enough of a workout, Jodi said we had to actually stay and move our bodies. She's never been that much fun. She led me to a piece of machinery the size of a Humvee with a control panel similar to that found in the cockpit of a commercial airplane. It was supposedly a treadmill. Before I could run on it, I had to enter my weight, speed, time, social security number, and mother's maiden name. Forty-five minutes later, the treadmill finally started and I began my jog. Once I got bored with the random facts being spewed out by the control panel, I started to look around, hoping to find something to amuse me. That's when I noticed what is by far the most exciting thing I've seen while running: a TV. And not just one. There were like eight TVs. How exciting is this? I can watch TV while I run nowhere! I can watch *Monday Night Football* or *Law & Order*—even fishing shows. Finally I'm able to accomplish something valuable while doing this pointless running! Now if I could only figure out how to strap one of those TVs to my head while I'm running the marathon. . . .

Now that I'm a gym-goer and a marathon-trainer and a 7 AM-on-a-Saturday awaker, many of my friends and family have expressed concern that I'm becoming a completely different person. They fear that a positive attitude and perky personality can't be too far off. I would like to calm those fears by assuring everyone that the Old Dawn is still alive and well. And she is loving all the ice cream and Tostitos Cheese Dip she is getting to eat without gaining any weight. And considering the fact that I've now run 115 miles without losing even one pound, I think it's fair to say that the Old Dawn is doing just fine.

CHAPTER *eight*
The Pain

If it hasn't been made clear by the previous chapters in this book, I would like to remind you that I am not a running professional of any sort. It should be okay for you to take my advice about most of the things I've discussed without wondering whether it will cause pain to you (spandex shorts) or others (short shorts). But when we start talking real pain instead of just psychological pain associated with bad fashion, I implore you to seek the advice of running or medical professionals before making any major decisions.

I'm not just saying this to avoid a lawsuit; I am saying it because there are a katrillion different injuries one can sustain while repeatedly pounding her body against hard surfaces like asphalt and park benches. There's no way I can list them all (nor would I want to, because some of them involve puss). Only a professional can tell you why you're in pain (it might have something to do with the hundreds of miles you're running) and what you should do to ease it (stop running and start drinking heavily). Plus, I really don't want to get sued.

● ● ●

LEVELS OF PAIN: A HELPFUL GUIDE TO UNDERSTANDING YOUR PAIN

LEVEL 1: "I need a nap."

LEVEL 2: "I need some Advil."

LEVEL 3: "I need to submerge my body in an ice bath."

LEVEL 4: "I need a stretcher."

LEVEL 5: "I need a full-body transplant (preferably transplanted with some sort of running machine)."

PREVENTION

Because of the katrillion different injuries you can sustain while training, I again offer you one blanket statement for avoiding injuries: Marathon training, like marathon running, is an endurance sport. Pushing yourself too hard or trying to go way beyond your physical limits is the surest way to get injured. If you're injured, the best way to stay injured is to continue running in hopes of "working out" the injury. Guess what? Injuries sustained from frequent high-impact exercise very rarely heal miraculously under continued exposure to frequent high-impact exercise. At least, I think that's what a professional might say.

One great way to avoid injury in the first place is to get the right shoes. Also, replace your shoes if you start to feel any leg and back pain later on in your training. This may mean that your shoes have lost their lust for life and it's time for new, excited shoes. Some people buy two pairs and rotate them throughout their training. This gives you time to break in both pairs early in training, so you don't have to go through that sometimes-uncomfortable process when the lengths of the runs are uncomfortable enough all by themselves.

When purchasing shoes, I highly recommend that you visit professional Shoe People. Most people working at running stores have the knowledge to help you pick the right shoes. Your shoes and the impact they have make them a key element in the health of the rest of your body. Starting off with good shoes is a huge step (pun totally intended) in getting you off on the right foot (I kill me) and will help you avoid running into any problems along the way (okay, I'm done now).

Other ways to avoid pain and injuries include proper hydration and stretching. Running injuries are unique in that most of the time the site of the injury is not the cause of the injury. Pain in the bottom of your foot can be helped by stretching your calf muscles; backaches can be aided by a change in stride; throbbing knees can relate to your hip. Proper hydration and stretching keep muscles healthy and happy, and they in turn provide comfort for the rest of your body. This is not to say that everything is going to be peachy friggin' keen, but those two little things will help you avoid a lot of pain and problems. That will give you plenty of time to deal with your multitude of other pains and problems. It's all about time management, really.

● ● ●

Journal Entry: WEEK 2
Runner's Hangover

I've begun to run every day. A mile here, two miles there, and up to four miles a couple of times. Every day a new part of my body aches. First it was my thighs, then my back, then my feet. The day after my first four-mile run, my body was very upset about my newfound love of running. My knees felt like Monica Lewinsky's after a job interview. It's been way too long since anyone had a good Monica Lewinsky joke. I'd laugh at my joke, but my stomach muscles are too sore.

Shortly after my body began falling apart, I got very sick. My head clogged up, and I felt like a pile of poo. I could barely keep my eyes open, and I could hardly muster the energy to walk down the stairs, much less run anywhere. I wasn't really sure what was going on. I had heard about this endorphin thing called a "Runner's High." Apparently, I had skipped this "Runner's High" and gone straight to the "Runner's Hangover." I've been told by many people who think they're my mother, and even the woman herself, that I should eat better. Apparently french fries and marshmallows aren't an appropriate training diet. Why do people have to be so negative?

So I've started to eat better and am drinking more water than can be healthy for a non-gilled life-form. And I'm feeling better. Unfortunately that means I have to start running again (my illness had given me a few days off). Next time I'm going to have to break an ankle to ensure a longer rest period.

But no, no, no. I can, I will, I am able. Stop trying to distract me.

TREATMENT

The key to dealing with pain during your training is being able
to distinguish between general holy-crap-since-when-does-this-
body-exercise pain and holy-crap-I-really-think-my-shin-just-
cracked-in-half pain. The former holy-crap pain occurs throughout training and eventually loses its shock value. It can usually be
eased by a killer combination of ice and Advil following a run.
Some Serious Runners actually take ice baths after their runs,
because ice is just that great for your weary muscles. This concept
starts making other parts of my body weary so I can't say that I've
tried it, but if you have a tub and the most productive icemaker
ever, you might want to give this a try. If you aren't looking to go
to the ice bath extreme, icing sore or swollen areas of your body is
a great postrun routine that will help a little in the holy-crap pain
area. Plastic bags of frozen peas make excellent ice packs and are
wonderfully moldable around things like knees and calf muscles.
Then when you're done, you can cook 'em up and make headway
on that healthy diet you should be eating.

It's important to remember that icing and Advil-ing are post-
run activities. Numbing pain before a run might seem fantastic in
theory but there's usually a reason you're in pain and that reason
is not going to go away simply because you're temporarily numb
to it. In fact, when the pain becomes un-numb you will need
to submerge yourself in an ice chest for three days to re-numb
your body that was pushed way past its limit during your Advil-
induced euphoria.

Warm baths or a Jacuzzi are always a good way to relax torn-up
muscles. But it's recommended that you hold off on hot-tubbing
until a couple hours after your run or until any swelling goes

down. Just chill out with the peas for a while. Maybe grab a head of lettuce and make a salad.

The major question one usually asks when pain arises is, "Can I keep training?" The answer often can be found by talking to one of those professionals I spoke of earlier. But I'll just say that a lot of marathon training is cut short because of injuries, most of which result from new runners overextending themselves. Yes, I know you're supposed to be on a schedule, and that if you divert from the schedule the world may end. But pushing your injured body is a great way to make sure you will fall completely off the schedule, with complete leg replacement as your only hope in returning.

If you have an injury, take it easy for a few days and give your body a chance to heal. Also, don't run on an injury in hopes of altering your running style to accommodate your pain. That's a sure way to pick up another injury, and then you'll be well on your way to a complete set. If you really want to exercise, try low-impact cross-training (e.g., swimming or cycling), as long as it doesn't aggravate the injury further.

For the numerous types of running-related injuries, there are even more ways to treat those injuries. If you begin to feel pain, I recommend talking to your coach and finding out his or her opinion. I also recommend going online to research your particular pain. You'll be amazed by what sort of remedies the Internet holds. Just to be safe, though, you'll probably want to consult a few sites to be sure the advice is sound before you start packing cow dung on your shins because an herbologist in Wichita recommended it.

The main principle of injury prevention is remembering to take your training slow and steady. A good training schedule, such as the one you can find on pages 6–13, is important in your training and should help you ease into running and avoid injuries. When reviewing the schedule, note all the activities on the schedule, not just the long runs. The long runs are important, but they're next to impossible if they aren't surrounded by the cross-training and smaller, easier runs. As I've mentioned before, your overall training is an effort to convince your body that it's a long-distance runner. Your body will not be convinced, nor will it be happy, if you are sporadic or overzealous in your training. So follow your training schedule, and try to steadily introduce your body to the world of running.

If you do this and your body still replies with a disgruntled injury, give it time. Believe me, you won't win any fight you pick with your fatigued body. No amount of wooing (via massages or pain medication) is going to help the situation if your body gets pushed into the serious injury category. So find a middle ground, where you agree to listen to your body when it sends you messages and it agrees to stay upright until you reach the marathon finish line. After that, all bets are off.

● ● ●

Journal Entry: WEEK 4
Eleven Miles

So I ran eleven miles this weekend. At 7 AM. As in before noon. On a Saturday. Eleven miles. Who runs eleven miles? What's the point? Why would a person ever, ever in her life need to run that far? You know a car? You push that little pedal on the right, and it takes you wherever you could want to go. It would probably take ten minutes to drive eleven miles. That's how long it takes me to run *one* mile. On a good day. On the first mile.

Who thought up this sport? And who thought to call it a sport? This is not a sport, this is a form of torture used to get important information from prisoners of war. "Tell me where the weapons of mass destruction are, or I'll make you run a marathon." "Oh please, please, no running, anything but running, I'll tell you anything you want to know." If you sent Chipper Jen in there with the threat, the entire Iraq situation would be taken care of in ten minutes flat.

I also must share that my toenail is turning black. Or maybe under my toenail is turning black. Either way, it isn't pretty, and I think I may be on my way to losing a nail. It is disgusting. But not completely unexpected. As soon as I started training for a marathon, people started coming out of the woodwork bearing tales of fallen toenails. I've been told that it's nothing to be alarmed about, that it's merely blood under my nail. Blood under my toenail actually seems slightly alarming. But honestly, it doesn't hurt and isn't supposed to start hurting any time soon; so I think I'll try to put it out of my mind and concentrate on more pressing

>>>

>>>

issues, like dehydration and the fact that I have committed to finishing a marathon.

That being said, I'm not sure how I'll react if the toenail falls off. But I know that I'll have to show Chipper Jen, because it will freak her out. And that alone is worth sacrificing a toenail for. Jen has taken her fear of losing toenails to an obsessive level. She has bought creams and polishes and nail files and nail strengtheners. She describes each product in great detail every time anyone mentions toenails. This amuses me no end. Her paranoia has been quite helpful. Every time she starts to ramble about the benefits of healthy eating and exercise, I just ask her, "Have your toenails fallen off yet?" and the ensuing panic attack usually derails her train of positive thinking. Cynicism trumps chipperness once again.

Part of your training is educating yourself about the body's muscles. Mainly you'll learn that you actually have muscles, knowledge acquired when these muscles announce their presence with jolts of pain during your months of training. I've never been more aware of my body parts than I was when they were all screaming at me every morning as I climbed/rolled/fell out of bed.

On the following page is space to list all your newfound muscles and the various pains that've manifested as they announce their places on your body.

● ● ●

MY MUSCLES AND HOW THEY ACHE

MUSCLE: _____

PAIN: _____

_____

MUSCLE: _____

PAIN: _____

_____

MUSCLE: _____

PAIN: _____

_____

MUSCLE: _____

PAIN: _____

_____

MUSCLE: _____

PAIN: _____

_____

MUSCLE: _____

PAIN: _____

_____

MUSCLE: _____

PAIN: _____

_____

MUSCLE: _____

PAIN: _____

_____

MUSCLE: _____

PAIN: _____

_____

Journal Entry: WEEK 12
I Heart Spandex

I ran eighteen miles this weekend. That was great fun. What did you do over the weekend? Did you go see a movie? Catch dinner with friends? Shop? Curl up on the couch and watch all ten years of *I Love the '80s* on VH1? In the time it would take you to do all those things *combined,* I ran eighteen miles. You think I'm kidding. Tragically, I am not.

We won't go into detail about how long it took me to run eighteen miles, because times and numbers are not the point. The point is that I'm not racing anyone but myself (and Oprah). I'm doing it for the journey, not the destination (pineapple drinks). And I'm everywoman (when life gets you down, just think about how things are going for Whitney; that ought to cheer you up).

But who am I kidding? The only people who say that times and numbers don't matter are the people with bad times and numbers. And I'm not so much everywoman as I am one woman who is desperately trying to locate her right kneecap. Yes, the big news of the weekend is that my right knee has officially left my body. But don't worry, it was kind enough to leave a sharp knife in its place.

The knee was last seen around Mile 11 of my nice little weekend jog. I don't know why I was surprised by its exit; it has been warning me for weeks that it wasn't happy with the current state of affairs. But did I heed this warning? Did I stop the running? No, I decided to run eighteen miles. I've always been a thinker.

>>>

>>>

My knee started hurting earlier in the week, during a nighttime run of only about six miles. (Note the word *only* before the words *six miles*. This is the kind of talk that drove the knee away.) I figured the change in temperature was responsible for my sudden knee pain. You see, the season of fall fell on Tuesday in Sacramento this year. It was a lovely twenty-four hour season. I thought maybe my body, and my knee, were in shock from running in ninety-degree weather one day and sixty-degree weather two days later.

I was told by a *Runner's World* subscriber that long running pants or tights might help my muscles stay warm in cool weather. You know what this means! Oh yes, it's true, it's exciting, it's . . . *more spandex!* Not just shorts, but long spandex. Double the coverage, double the excitement. I didn't think anything could look worse than my spandex shorts. I was so, so wrong.

Spandex provides the unique fashion style of body parts being held against their will. And these body parts do not give up without a fight. The more spandex covers, the more my jiggling body is longing to be free. I'm not a big fan of tight clothes, so I decided to throw baggy shorts on over my spandex. Questionable fashion? Yes. My spandexed butt out for the world to see? No.

With a new Running Outfit ready for its inaugural run, I hit the bike trail around noon. Other people training for the marathon hit the trail around 7 AM. On Saturday. Now that it's cool all day long, I can find no logic whatsoever in Saturday morning runs. Many runners say that it's easier to run when you're with a group. I do not agree. Unless a member of the running team is planning to carry me, there's nothing to

>>>

>>>

be gained by running with a group. Besides, I only get to run with the group for two minutes before they run off and leave me alone with my twenty-minute-mile pace. They are not team players.

But when you get down to it, running is about as individual a sport as you're gonna find. There are no team members, there are no opponents, there are no time-outs to talk over strategy with the other players. There's just you and miles of open road ahead. I don't know if I can adequately explain how much running it takes to run eighteen miles. And while your body is doing all this work, your brain is left with little to do. This leads to boredom like you would not believe.

Imagine sitting in a chair staring at the wall for four hours. You can't read a book, you can't watch TV, you can't do a crossword puzzle. You just stare and think. You wouldn't be able to do it because people aren't meant to do such things. That's why god gave us the Internet and cable and even other human beings (in case the power goes out). After Month 2 of this running thing, I had run out of thoughts. Even my radio isn't keeping my brain entertained anymore. After a couple hours, I completely tune out the music. And for good reason. I've been listening to the same songs over and over again for three months. Whenever the radio announcer says, "Here's a new one from . . ." I get so excited I nearly giggle.

Thank god I like a diversity of music, so I can switch between rock and rap and country and love songs. But the songs that cross several genres play on every station at least twenty-eight times a day. If I hear matchbox twenty's "Unwell" one more time, I swear on a pineapple drink I may myself become very, very unwell.

>>>

>>>

In an effort to stimulate my brain I've begun listening to talk radio. I will listen to some guy go on and on about stock portfolios or spew politics that I am completely against just so I can give my brain something to focus on for a while. And I just can't get enough of that Paul Harvey, "The Rest of the Story" guy. I know the rest of so many stories, it's ridiculous. Where does he find these stories? Do you ever think he just makes them up? He's gotta be like 110 years old by now. So who's gonna have the guts to call him a liar? "Paul, I really don't think Einstein came up with the $E = mc^2$ thing during a game of Scrabble . . . "

I just realized how boring the last paragraph was. But during an eighteen-mile run, that paragraph is jam-packed with excitement. Add that to my baggy shorts, long spandex, and limp, and I think I've officially become a dork.

But there is good news. Today is November 14. Do you know what happens one month from today? On December 14, I run a marathon. And do you know what happens December 15? I get out of the hospital, *and then*, despite the wishes of my fans and the spandex industry and matchbox twenty, I hang up my running shoes, put on some slippers, and take a nap. And there will be no rest of the story for Paul Harvey to report. Unless he wants to make up a story. In which case I would like to beat P. Diddy's marathon time and look like J.Lo while doing it.

One more month, one more month, one more month. . . .

CHAPTER *nine*
The Fundraising

If you're running a marathon for a good cause (not that a toned butt isn't a good enough cause), you will not only be taking on the challenge of training but also that of prying money out of people's wallets. Sometimes it will seem as if running twenty-six miles is nothing in comparison to asking people for money. 'Cause people love their money.

Raising money for a worthy cause can be a significant reason to begin training. But the prospect of taking money from worthy people should never be the reason to quit training. Different teams have different fundraising minimums, which can increase as the coolness factor of the marathon location increases. I had the choice of running a marathon in Arizona or Hawaii. To go to Hawaii I had to raise a $1,000 more. I knew this was going to be difficult, but I also knew that a marathon without pineapple drinks and beaches at the finish line was not the marathon for me. Some people may be more motivated by logic than I and therefore may choose a marathon that requires the least amount of fundraising, not the one with best access to beaches.

Before you pick a team to train with, put out feelers to people you think may contribute large sums to your cause. This will ease some of your reservations about your fundraising commitment. If you're lucky like me, you'll have very supportive family members who pledge large sums of money once they wake up from their shock-induced coma caused by your marathon-training announcement. "You know, I could have just sent you to Hawaii for the amount of money I donated to your fundraising," my mother said. "And then I wouldn't have had to go through all that crazy training and hard work and losing of my kneecaps," I pointed out. To which she replied, "Yeah, but then again, I wouldn't have been able to get the tax write-off if I just sent you there."

On the off chance you don't have a mother who is willing to trade your pain and suffering for her tax breaks, I offer you a detailed breakdown of other people who might financially support the removal of your kneecaps.

FRIENDS AND FAMILY

Friends and family will be the easiest to get money out of. These people like you. Well, at least your friends probably do. The family can go either way. But family is genetically obligated to see you during holidays; so if nothing else, they might pledge just to avoid being the one holdout sitting around the Thanksgiving table. That's a good way to lose dibs on the stuffing and be stuck with only the questionable-looking canned cranberry sauce.

If you're training with a big group, such as the National AIDS Marathon or Leukemia & Lymphoma Society's Team in Training, it will most likely give you various fundraising materials. Groups often provide a letter/email template of a prewritten letter that lets you insert your name in certain places and send it out. I'm sure these letters work for some people, and if you want to give them a shot I say go for it. But I didn't think a prewritten letter provided enough of my own personality to interest my friends and family (they're a tough crowd). I entered the marathon for personal reasons and because I had very much lost my mind. I wanted to convey these facts in my fundraising pleas, which a prewritten letter couldn't adequately do.

Instead I sent periodic emails to friends and family updating them on my steady run toward a marathon and the emergency room. These emails included stories and pictures from my training, as well as a link to my fundraising web page. Some people send their fundraising letters via snail mail, but I felt like email was the best way to reach people. It's free, as opposed to the cost of paper, envelopes, and stamps. Email's biggest benefit was that it gave me the ability to have conversations with friends and family about my training after they received my electronic updates. After I sent updates, I'd hear back from people encouraging me, relating to me, or just mocking me. I'd email back and forth with them, which often led to donations, yes, but also provided a lot of moral support for me throughout my training. There's nothing like a "Girl, you've lost your damn mind" email to keep you motivated.

Another benefit of email is that it's easy for recipients to forward your email updates on to someone else they think might be interested in your story or your cause. I often receive email replies from random people who had been forwarded my updates and wanted to donate to my fundraising. You never know who might be moved by your story, and email is definitely the fastest and most effective way to reach those people.

Keep in mind the importance of repetition. Repetition, repetition, repetition. Friends and family care about you and will want to help out in anything you are doing, amazingly stupid or otherwise. But surprisingly enough, they actually have lives of their own. Although you may find it impossible to forget the hell you're enduring for the sake of a toned butt (and charity), friends often need to be reminded of the hell you're enduring for the sake of prying money out of their wallets.

Regular email updates are a great way to stay in contact with your friends and family and to gently nudge them into donating. A lot of people really want to donate, but then the thought exits their minds as soon as they open the next email that is offering specials on pharmaceuticals or heart-warming poems celebrating Beautiful Women's Month. If you send out a few more updates on your training, then eventually you may receive a friendly if jumbled response: "I'm all stocked up on OxyContin and it's been Beautiful Women's Month for three years straight, so I'm ready to donate to my dear friend's painful training. It's too bad that she's lost the use of her joints, but damn if that isn't entertaining to me and worth a little donation. And that's not just the OxyContin talking."

I know not everyone is like me and is blessed with the ability to write on and on ad nauseam about herself (is narcissism an ability?). But you're going through one of the most challenging, painful, exhilarating, and butt-toning experiences of your life. I know you can come up with a paragraph or two about your training to put in an email. If you're at a loss, consult the handy journal you're keeping because I told you to. There's bound to be a funny or touching story there. Your emails don't have to be filled with prose as brilliant as mine (yes, I think narcissism is an ability), they just need to be filled with you. Then they will resonate with your friends and family and with their checkbooks.

One thing to remember when sending email updates/pleas: Cast your net wide. Do not hesitate to put everyone on the list. If you have their email address, send them an update. You never know who is going to end up feeling inspired to donate to your cause, and increasing your odds is always a wise idea. Also, be prepared to be shocked by where your donations end up coming from. The people you expect to hand you wads of cash will usually be the ones who give a $10 donation. The biggest donations will usually come from the most unlikely places. And if you're anything like me, you'll find that people's generosity becomes a major reason for continuing your training. If people are willing to part with their hard-earned cash on the faith that you will actually complete a marathon, it's very difficult to let them down.

ACQUAINTANCES

These are people you'll never sit down to Thanksgiving dinner with and who feel no obligation to give you any money in exchange for dibs on stuffing. You may have to work a little harder to wrestle money from them. But you're in the best shape of your life, so you are definitely ready for some wrestling.

I found that acquaintances usually want something in return for their money. Your blood, sweat, and tears aren't enough for them; they need to feel as if they're getting something tangible for their money. This requires a little creativity on your part, but you've already figured out ways to navigate a sports bra, apply BODYGLIDE, and eat a PowerBar all at the same time—you, my dear, are nothing if not creative.

Think of something you can, in effect, sell to these people. If you're artistic, you can sell the things you make—paintings, needlepoint, handmade cards, lapel pins, or knitted scarves. Do not attempt this if you're not artistic, unless you have an adorable child who you can say is the actual artist behind the creations.

I'm an artistic person. But I was also a person trying to juggle 8,453 things during my training. So whipping up twenty paintings just wasn't fitting into my schedule. Instead, I chose to turn to another talent: eating. No, I didn't win any prize money from any sort of eating contest (only because I just now thought of that), but I knew I wasn't the only person out there who enjoyed eating. So I decided to turn that enjoyment into fundraising.

I called my favorite local Mexican restaurant and spoke to the manager about hosting a fundraising night there. We picked a night when business is slow. I distributed flyers and emails to friends and acquaintances inviting them to come eat dinner at the restaurant on that night, and the restaurant would then donate a percentage of its receipts to my charity. It was a win for the restaurant because I brought them business, a win for me because I raised money toward my fundraising, and a win for the people who got to eat good food for a good cause because everyone likes good food.

You can plan several events like this over the course of your training and they can bring in a nice chunk of change. You can also do a variation of this at local bars or pool halls, and work out an agreement that a percentage of the receipts you bring in are donated. Kinda like the arrangement bars often have with bands. But instead of staging a musical act, you'll be reenacting your sports bra/BODYGLIDE/PowerBar feat, which should end up being equally entertaining.

Journal Entry: WEEK 8
Hooters

Chipper Jen and I are getting quite creative in our fundraising efforts. This weekend we washed cars in an attempt to raise money. To make the event as fun and as lucrative as possible, Chipper Jen and I wore Hooters T-shirts. No, neither of us is a current or previous employee of that organization. I'm a bit of a tomboy and bought the shirt as a joke, because I'm pretty much the opposite of a Hooters girl. But, as it turns out, I actually have hooters, so why not use them to try to raise money for a good cause? My momma always said, "If you got it, flaunt it." Or maybe that was my friend Marcus. He's a tall black man, and she's a short white woman, so you understand the confusion. Either way, I'd like to flaunt them while I still got 'em, because I'm pretty sure that all of this running is going to leave them somewhere in the vicinity of my knees by December. That might be more information than you needed. But let's just say, there's a reason why you never see large-chested women finishing marathons first. They've been beaten to death by their breasts around Mile 5. It ain't pretty.

But what isn't pretty while running actually turned out to be lucrative while soaping down dirty cars. Chipper Jen and I set up our car wash at a gas station early Saturday morning. We came equipped with CAR WASH signs in hand, Hooters shirts on bodies, and sponges a soakin'. Within minutes, cars started coming in. And they didn't stop for three solid hours.

I stationed Chipper Jen on the corner with the CAR WASH sign and her natural tendency to bounce and smile and lure people to her warm personality. On

>>>

>>>

Saturday, her warm personality became even more al-luring because it was hidden beneath a tight Hooters shirt. All morning, we heard tires screech and would look up to see a woman smacking a man upside the head. Fundraising for a good cause really has a way of bringing people together, doesn't it?

While Chipper Jen caused traffic accidents and divorc-es on the corner, I worked diligently on cleaning the cars. I was constantly surprised by how much money people gave me to wash their cars, ten to twenty dol-lars every time. One nice, older gentleman brought three different cars and paid us twenty dollars each time. What a generous man.

Toward the end of the car wash, one of my friends who was helping out pointed at my chest and said, "Are we having a wet T-shirt contest? 'Cause I think you're winning." I looked down at my shirt and realized that my very tight, very white shirt was also very wet as well. It became clear that not only was I washing cars, I was also giving them quite a show. I stopped to think about whether I was embarrassed by this, but my thinking was interrupted by another friend announc-ing that we'd raised nearly $500 in three hours. I then proceeded to spray myself with water and get back to work. I also asked the gas station owner if his corner was available every weekend. I might just come back and do some fundraising for my rent.

COMPLETE STRANGERS

Sure, you've never met these people before, but they are just sitting around waiting for you to do something so they can hand you some of their money. So go do something already!

The way Chipper Jen and I reached out to complete strangers was by having a car wash. Two car washes earned us a ridiculous amount of money—$800—in a very short time.

The car wash also allowed us to call on some of our friends and family members who wanted to support our cause but weren't in a financial situation to donate large sums of money. Instead they helped us out by donating their time washing cars and collecting large sums of money from complete strangers. If you hang out with rich friends, you might be able to skip the whole car wash thing and just get money directly from the friends. Unfortunately, I don't have rich friends. So I was made to wear a Hooters shirt and wash cars. That reminds me; I need to get more rich friends.

A garage sale can also be an easy way to raise money. Complete strangers go *crazy* for garage sales. I can't say I totally understand the mentality of someone who wakes up at 5 AM on Saturday to peruse other people's discarded items. But I can say that it's a good way to raise cash. Call on those not-rich friends of yours to go through their piles of pointless crap (it doesn't take wealth to accumulate pointless crap); then they can give the stuff to you, and you can sell it to people wanting to buy pointless crap. It is the circle of life, really. Or the circle of crap, as it were.

Like I said, cast your net wide on all things fundraising. It's always better to have too many donations than too few. And remember that everyone and their mother is raising money for something (*especially* mothers, "You wanna buy a bin of popcorn

to help support my child's Frisbee team? What about some wrap-
ping paper to help buy the school a new flagpole?"). Be creative,
and make sure as many people as possible know that you are training for a marathon and are raising money. Remember that you
and the cause you are raising money for are both doing good
things, so don't ever feel guilty about raising money. (When you
are standing at the bottom of a flight of stairs, trying to muster the
resolve to climb them, go ahead and tell people why. They may
give you some money, or at the very least a piggy-back ride.)

THE PREWRITTEN LETTER

I've included one of those prewritten letters I mentioned earlier. I
still recommend you avoid them and write email updates in your
own voice, because the people receiving them know you and will
know the difference between your voice and the voice of some
sarcastic writer who enjoys talking about herself to no end. If
you need to, though, use this letter as a jumping-off point. I've
included space where you can fill in your own stories and info.

Hey everyone,

I am writing with yet another dispatch from the frontlines of marathon training. The training is going well, and
I want to assure you all that I am still alive despite the
grueling mileage we've been running lately. Our team is
now running up to XX miles at a time, and that number
goes up every week as we inch (or mile) our way closer
to 26.2.

All this running is difficult to do but it sure does provide
some great stories. *(Insert a funny or touching story here. Most
of the people you are writing to are not runners nor do they ever
intend to be, so try to make the story relatable to people who*

have no idea what the hell GU is. Not that you can't talk about GU. In fact talk about GU and tell how extremely bizarre it is to eat strawberry-flavored hair gel at Mile 15.)

I've attached a picture of myself and some of my running buddies from our XX-mile run the other day. Some of you may want to print this out as concrete proof that your favorite nonrunner is in fact training for a marathon.

I want to thank everyone for their support during my training. Your kind (and sometimes funny) words have helped a lot, and I feel lucky to have such great friends. As you know, I am doing this marathon as a fundraiser for *(fill in the organization's name);* and if any of you are interested in helping me reach my fundraising goal, I would really appreciate it. You can email me for more info on donating, or you can go directly to my fundraising web page: www.fillintheURL.com. *(Most major fundraising organizations will provide you with a personalized fundraising page that allows people to donate online.)*

Thanks again for your words and your donations. Both help me as I pound the pavement and slowly make my way to marathon glory.

Talk soon,

(Your name)

THE
∧ PAYOFF

CHAPTER *ten*

The Mentality

There's no underestimating the importance of preparing yourself mentally as well as physically for your marathon. Running a successful race relies heavily on your state of mind. It's easy to feel intimidated by the ridiculous number of miles ahead of you; but honestly, they aren't any more ridiculous than the miles behind you. What's another twenty-six when you've run *hundreds?* I mean, come on.

It's not like you just happened upon this marathon, like you were out window-shopping, saw a marathon going on, and decided it might be fun to jump right in. (Don't laugh, some people actually do this. These idiots realize pretty quickly that window-shopping might be the most strenuous activity they are trained to take on.) If you're a window-shopper, I say that it's perfectly okay for you to be intimidated by this marathon. But that isn't the case. The case is that you have been diligently training for this day for months. You have dramatically altered your lifestyle and your sanity levels and slowly but surely molded yourself into the fierce running machine that you are today.

So why do you feel like you're about to puke or cry at any moment? Because THIS IS IT!!! THE MOMENT YOU'VE BEEN WAITING FOR!!! And other caps-locked exclamations. It's hard not to be slightly intimidated by an event that has been built up like the Second Coming of Christ (or Elvis) for the last five months. Everything you have done has lead to this very day. It's all quite dramatic. And it all has quite a way of messing with your head.

Speaking of your head, let's work a little logic into your panic attack. Logically, mathematically, you have to believe that you are ready for this run. You have to think back over the training you've put yourself through, and you have to realize that it wasn't just some form of cruel torture that masochistic running coaches came up with to pass the time. It was actually all done to prepare you for what you're going to encounter during your marathon. (The torture part will provide a particularly handy reference point.)

You've spent months figuring out exactly what food works with your stomach before a run, exactly when you'll stop and walk, exactly which color hat complements your eye color. You've been doing a lot of work so that you'll know what the hell to do during your marathon. Now it's time to trust yourself and your training and your hat color and attack your marathon with confidence and pride. Can I get a "Go Girl!"?

Journal Entry: **WEEK 13**
I Can, I Will, I'm Oprah

With less than a month to go until my first/last marathon, I have an announcement to make. No, I am not dropping the marathon in favor of entering a hula contest in Hawaii. Although that doesn't sound like a bad idea. I must say, I do look stunning wearing a coconut bikini and a grass skirt. Yet I digress.

>>>

>>>

My announcement is this: I've had a drastic change of attitude these past few weeks. I've gone from not particularly caring that it's going to take me eight hours to finish 26.2 miles to particularly caring that it is going to take me eight hours to finish 26.2 miles. This is no longer an acceptable timeframe for me. What inspired my change of heart? Well, it wasn't just one thing, it was a combination of things. The first thing that got this attitude ball rolling was the thing that inspires all of life's major changes: Oprah Winfrey.

No, I didn't see a special Oprah show that inspired me to become a new me and live my best life or any of that crap. I learned that Oprah Winfrey finished a marathon in four hours and thirty minutes. That is three hours and thirty minutes faster than the eight hours I'm anticipating it will take me. This bothers me more than I can explain. I simply cannot get my butt kicked by Oprah in a marathon. In book reading or meditating or private jet buying, she can kick my butt. But not running.

You see, I'm pretty competitive. I don't like to lose. At all. In fact, I rarely play if I think I'm gonna lose. But my competitiveness had never become a factor in this running thing. I kept wondering why I didn't particularly care that I was the slowest runner in the history of the world. Normally being the worst would bother me quite a bit. But I just didn't care. And not in that I-don't-care!-throw-something-down-on-the-ground-and-storm-off sort of way. I really was okay with being horrible.

I think this is because this running thing isn't a real sport. In real sports you have something you're going after—a ball or a basket or other players' shins. This motivates you, you want to get that ball or make that

>>>

>>>

basket or see that player on the ground. But with running, the only real goal is to not die. The only time I feel motivated is when I see a water fountain ahead. When I get to the water fountain and it spits out only enough water to hydrate an ant, I am then motivated to kick it repeatedly. These are the emotions I need in a sport.

When you're running twenty-six miles, there isn't that sense of immediacy that you get in a sudden-death overtime or at the bottom of the ninth, two outs, full count. There's still the possibility of sudden death, but even that's probably not gonna happen for another eight friggin' miles. So I just bounce along, going nowhere, not able to slide tackle anyone.

But now that has all changed. I've found someone to slide tackle, so to speak. And that someone is Oprah. I don't harbor any ill feelings toward her at all. I love Oprah. Everyone loves Oprah. Oprah even loves Oprah. But if Oprah can do this, I can too. Look at the stats: She was forty years old and had years of weight fluctuations, weird diets, and bad hair to contend with when she ran. I am twenty-five, have always been in relatively good shape, and only had really bad hair in seventh grade. I should be able to do this.

And I guess that's where the change of attitude came in. Since Day 1, I've never had high expectations for this whole running thing. And as Oprah will tell you every day on TV and twice a page in her magazine, if you have mediocre expectations then you're going to have mediocre results. So as of today, my expectations have changed. I'm no longer simply accepting the fact that I'm going to spend the better part of a workday running a marathon.

>>>

Oprah was older than I am, heavier than I am, and wore more spandex than I do—and she finished a marathon in four hours and thirty minutes. I'm young, I'm in shape, and I'm aiming for five hours, maybe five and a half. I've changed my attitude, but I'm not delusional. I've got less than a month to live my best life. What do you want from me? Oprah will definitely still beat me, but at least she'll beat me while I'm actually trying, instead of bouncing along looking for a water fountain to kick. So, I'm gonna play, even though I know I'm probably not gonna win. Because I'm a changed woman! Someone get Maya Angelou, and let's have us a group hug!

Unfortunately, one does not get into shape with attitude alone. This realization was a temporary setback in the living of my new life. I know I need to work out more and push myself harder and be everywoman who roars. But I don't really like moving, remember? Yes, I forgot about that during my attitude change. But never fear, I've got a secret weapon that even Oprah with her billions of dollars didn't have. I've got Chipper Jen. Yes I do. And Chipper Jen is ever so excited about my change of heart. Mostly because it involved me telling her that I needed her to kick my ass and make me go to the gym and make me work out. These are very exciting things for Jen.

Jen is so excited, in fact, that she has enlisted the help of Jodi, another chipper, gym-going friend. The two have figured out a shared custody arrangement: Jodi gets to kick my butt at the gym on Mondays and Wednesdays; Jen takes me on Fridays and Sundays. I don't know who gets me for the major holidays.

Their main goal is to get me on a gym machine other than a treadmill. You see, I haven't been doing much

>>>

besides running for my training. Now granted, I've run *a lot*. But apparently there are other muscles in your body besides the ones in your legs. Who knew? Well, now I know. How? Because every single one of those muscles hurts the day after my first workout with Jodi. We did weights and lifts and pushes and rolls and sit-ups. Well, I tried to do sit-ups. For some reason I am physically incapable of doing them. It turns out that any exercise that begins with me lying down is not really gonna get too far. Hopefully my trainers will take note of this.

I also learned another little stretchy thing that is supposed to help my knee find its way back to my body. Apparently the problem with my knee involves something called the IT band that runs from my hip to my knee. The old me would have attached another couple of letters to the beginning of that acronym, but I'm a changed woman and will just tell you about the stretch (you should really try it): Okay, first, stand up. Good job. Then put the outside of your right foot on your left thigh, like you're crossing your legs. Then squat down like you are sitting. Do you feel that? Oh wait. I forgot to tell you to hold on to a tree. Okay, get up off the ground. Now, hold on to a tree and put your foot up and then sit on your imaginary seat. Now, do you feel that? That's your IT band screaming out for you to sit in a real chair.

That's just a sample of what I feel every step of my eight-hour run. But there's usually at least one person doing a ridiculous stretch like that every mile. And the visual of spandex and squatting and pain entertains me more than I can explain. We might have Maya Angelou write a poem about it after our hug.

HOLY MOOD SWINGS, BATMAN

Like many first-timers, I experienced quite a few pre-marathon jitters. Well, they actually felt less like jitters and more like an overwhelming sense of dread and panic. This panic led to many pre-marathon fears, both legitimate and completely ridiculous. Then a few seconds later the panic would be replaced by a sense of excitement about my impending 26.2 miles. It was a fun experiment in the number of emotions one body can experience simultaneously. Usually this is referred to as PMS; but in this case, the clinical term is HCIHRM (Holy Crap I Have to Run a Marathon).

MY MARATHON FEARS (THE CONDENSED VERSION)

- What if I'm not ready?
- What if I fail?
- What if I pass out? Will the people who find me know to take me directly to the nearest beach with pineapple drinks?
- What if I get lost?
- What if Chipper Jen finishes and returns to the hotel without me? Will there be any pineapple drinks left by the time I get there?
- How high was I to have ever thought this would be a good idea?
- Can I be high while running the race?
- What if I do permanent damage to my knee?
- Would that ensure that I'd never have to run again?
- What if I'm the last person to cross the finish line?
- What if I'm not ready?
- What if I fail?

MY MARATHON EXCITEMENT

- Crossing the finish line.
- The pineapple drinks after I finish.
- The last time I'm ever required to run in my life.
- Running with 25,000 people (24,990 of whom may be running ahead of me).
- Setting a goal and achieving it.
- The amount of food I will consume after I'm done with the marathon.
- Finishing something I started.

As you set off on your marathon, keep reminding yourself that you're ready and that just by starting this marathon you've succeeded. Also remember that once you've finished, the words "long run" can once again refer to any distance greater than that which lies between your recliner and the refrigerator. This is the stuff that will keep you motivated and moving for the entire 26.2 miles.

Use the space on the following page to jot down some of your fears about your marathon, as well as the reasons why you have nothing to fear because you are a running machine, fueled by dreams, desires, and your couch that awaits you after the finish line.

● ● ●

FEAR: _____

WHY THIS IS RIDICULOUS: _____

_____

FEAR: _____

WHY THIS IS RIDICULOUS: _____

_____

FEAR: _____

WHY THIS IS RIDICULOUS: _____

_____

FEAR: _____

WHY THIS IS RIDICULOUS: _____

_____

FEAR: _____

WHY THIS IS RIDICULOUS: _____

_____

FEAR: _____

WHY THIS IS RIDICULOUS: _____

_____

FEAR: _____

WHY THIS IS RIDICULOUS: _____

_____

Now, on the following page, list some things you're excited about as you get closer to your marathon. Remember to actually get excited, maybe even a little giddy about the road ahead. Even though taking on 26.2 miles is a bit overwhelming, it's also very exhilarating. And if you get yourself pumped up about it, those positive emotions will help you tackle that looming marathon.

I'M EXCITED BECAUSE . . .

_____

_____

_____

_____

_____

_____

_____

_____

_____

_____

Journal Entry: WEEK 15
Oh, Crap!

Oh crap, oh crap, oh crap! I have to run a marathon in less than a week. Seriously. In like four days. 26.2 miles. In a row. You know that new attitude thing I talked about back when I was starting to get pumped about running this thing: I was gonna run a marathon and I was gonna do well and I was going to be every-woman. Well, that was before I realized I actually have to run a marathon in less than a week. Oh crap.

This marathon had become just another thing I was *gonna* do. There are a lot of things I'm *gonna* do *someday*. I may travel to Europe; I may have kids; I may touch my toes. *Someday*. Not today, not tomorrow, and definitely not on Sunday. There's no way I can touch my toes by Sunday.

>>>

>>>

But somehow it's gone from being a thing I talked about at parties to something I actually have to do. I don't wanna do a marathon. I just want to keep going to parties and talking about it. "Yeah, I'm gonna do a marathon. When? Oh, you know, down the road a little. And someday I might touch my toes, too."

What the hell was I thinking when I said I would do this? Obviously I wasn't thinking. There was no thinking involved whatsoever. I got a postcard with happy people running and I thought, *I can do that.* I was wrong, so so so so wrong. You know who I blame? The people who make those little "Horrific Life Story in Two Minutes" segments that always air before major sporting events. They feature someone competing who almost died, is dying, or has just lost a loved one. These athletes continue to compete even in the face of adversity. They work hard, push themselves, and find a way past the heartache and hurt of a difficult life to glory and victory and usually a lot of sweat.

No matter how cheesy the segments, I'm inevitably wiping my eyes at the end of the two minutes of slow-motion running and inspirational music. And if the subject ends up winning his event—I'm done. I'm crying like a baby, "Just look at that guy! His mom, dad, sister, dog, cat, and best friend all died when he was two. He raised himself, growing up on the streets, and he donated several organs to sick people. Now he's just won the gold medal in the balance beam! So everything's okay! Isn't that a great story?!"

And there's the problem: I'm a sucker for a good story. So when I heard the stories of the stroke victims who've finished marathons or saw the videos of the

>>>

>>>

happy people finishing their marathons in tears, I was hooked. And then the whole thing was a fundraiser for a good cause? Sign me up! Fast-forward four months and now all the stories have faded away. Now there's just me and twenty-six miles and one bad knee. I think I may be the first athlete in history who cries *before* the race.

What am I gonna do? Seriously, I just don't know. I had been training pretty well following my Oprah-induced desire to compete. But the training came to a screeching halt when I caught the flu. For about five days I was feeling like a general pile of poo and decided to hold off on exercising because, well, exercising sucks even when I feel great. What were the odds it was gonna go well when I already felt horrible? Not good.

After sleeping and self-medicating for a few days, I decided to complete my total body healing by going for a sports massage. I was told that a good sports massage would help my aching knee and convince it to stay on my body until next Sunday afternoon at least. So, I signed up for the massage and went to my appointment ready to be relaxed and renewed. Little did I know that the words "sports massage" are athletes' code for "stretch your body from one side of the room to the other and then repeat six times." Oh my.

My poor body did not know what hit it. It was expecting one of those waterfall machines and some Zen music. Instead what it got was, "Inhale as I push your knee into your chest. Okay, now exhale as I pull your leg back and try to touch your toe to the top of your head." 'Cause apparently exhaling makes that little stretch just a piece of cake. My body was pretzeled into various configurations throughout my "sports not-really-a massage," but the conversation with my

>>>

>>>

masseur seemed to keep my mind off of the fact that both of my feet were behind my head.

What conversation could have been that interesting? Well, my masseur told me he'd been a runner all his life. He started running when he was a kid 'cause he always tried to catch butterflies and would run miles after them. (I imagine he also ran away from the bullies who picked on him for collecting butterflies, yet I digress.) He loves running; he's a great runner; he showed me his wall of running trophies. And then he mentioned how he had never run a marathon and never intended to. "I don't think I could do it." "What?!" Inhale, knee up. ". . . But you love running!" Exhale, leg disconnected from body. "I know," he said, "but it just seems like too much." "Oh, we are gonna need to do a *lot* more stretching of my body."

After all my body parts were returned to their intended positions, I tried out my newly stretched knee on a short run. Surely it will be all better after being stretched for an hour; surely an hour sports massage can erase months' worth of damage I've done to my unsuspecting knee. If you don't see where this is going then you're in the same stretching position that I was in—the one in which your head is up your ass. I'm actually quite good at that one.

Shockingly enough, my knee was not cured and still feels like someone is taking a hammer to it with every step. But at least I'm not dramatic. Because that would be bad.

So what I've got going for me as I enter my marathon is (1) an abnormal amount of phlegm in too many parts of my head and chest, (2) only one functioning knee, and (3) a really positive attitude. Did I mention I'm screwed?

>>>

>>>

This is where my friends come in. I went to a marathon prep thingy the other night and a very excited runner told us to dedicate each mile to someone we care about because this will help us get through the miles. She recommended that we write people's names on our wrists or shirts or something. I don't know, I wasn't really paying attention, because I know that as much as I love my family and friends, their names written on my friggin' arm aren't going to help me much around Mile 21. Their names written on the side of a taxicab would be a different matter.

But I had another idea, one that might actually work for me. I asked my friends to write a sentence or two to cheer me on, the more sarcastic and off-color the better. I'm going to print these sentences out, laminate them individually, and then put them in my pouch. Then, as I get more and more tired and pissed off and unhappy during the run, I can simply reach into my pouch and pull out, "Try exercising while lactating and you'll have a whole new appreciation for your breasts." (Someone really contributed that sentence to my pouch.) Then I'll smile a little and pin the sentiment to my shirt. By the end of the marathon I'll have what looks like a grass skirt of jokes and inspirational quotes. And I'll be ready for my pineapple drinks. It will be adorable.

In other news, I have reached my fundraising minimum! How exciting is that? And no kidneys were sacrificed in the money-raising efforts. Even more exciting. I'm grateful to everyone who paid me to endure the pain of running twenty-six miles. I have given them my personal guarantee that I will cross the finish line. I am not guaranteeing that it won't be on a moped.

"INSPIRING" QUOTES THAT GOT ME THROUGH MY MARATHON

From Mark Twain:

- "Under certain circumstances, profanity provides a relief denied even to prayer."

From my friends:

- "All this and you haven't lost a pound???"
- "Right about Mile 16, when you're wishing like all hell that you were smart enough to stick cab fare in your GU pouch, keep saying over and over again, 'Just keep running, just keep running, running . . . running . . . just keep running.'"
- "Have an umbrella drink for me once you get discharged from the hospital."
- "Cheer up, things can get worse . . . and by the next mile, they will!"
- "You are flying hundreds of miles to beautiful islands and you are whining about a little pain in the knee?"
- "Gatorade, right hand, drink. Water, left hand, toss on head to keep cool. Warning: At Mile 21, do not confuse the two!!"
- "I am lying down right now, watching TV. What are you doing?"
- "Got spandex?"
- *"Don't* break a leg."
- "Look on the bright side—you're running in Hawaii."
- "We love you, bad knees and all."
- "Run, Dawn, run!"
- "You can't catch me!!!!!!" (That was Chipper Jen.)
- "I am closer than you are!!" (Another gem from Jen.)

- "Bladders and gravity may lead to depravity,
  so here's hoping your runs are all dry,
  if the road's a bit drafty,
  you'll have to be crafty.
  or you'll be wiping that stuff from your eye."

CHAPTER *eleven*
The Marathon

So here we are. The end of the training road. Which is actually the beginning of your marathon road. How friggin' poetic can you get? You have bled, sweated, and teared up for the past five months, and now you are ready to do it for the next 26.2 miles. Isn't this a great sport?

The most important thing to remember is that you are totally prepared for the twenty-six miles that lie before you. It's easy to get overwhelmed by the mix of excitement and fear you will feel in the days and hours leading up to your big day. Nothing I say can completely calm those feelings. That's okay, because this marathon is a big deal and is worth a few mood swings. But try not to let those emotions get so out of hand that they affect your ability to tackle your race head on. Below I list things you can do before and after the marathon to make the trip to the finish line a little more enjoyable. But I repeat, you have already done most of the work to prepare for this day.

PRE-MARATHON

The week before the marathon is by far the best week of training. Look at your training schedule, and you'll see an absolutely beautiful repetition of the word "rest" throughout the week. If that wasn't enough, this week you start carbo-loading in preparation for your big event. Rest and carbo-loading—this is my kind of training program.

The week before your marathon you are officially in self-preservation mode. Don't do anything that might hurt your chances of starting or finishing your marathon: Don't try new foods; don't do strenuous exercise (if you aren't taking advantage of the Rest Days listed on your training calendar, then I really have taught you nothing); and make every effort to avoid anyone who even looks like they might be sick. The last thing you need is a virus to go along with your dehydration and heatstroke on marathon day.

For three days before your marathon you will start becoming very friendly with carbohydrates and water. This is when you give your body the fuel it will need to keep you upright for the entirety of the marathon. During those days, add one to two extra servings of carbohydrates to your diet. (Seriously, best week ever.) You can also add an extra serving of protein, which will help repair your fatigued muscles. As much fun as all this resting and carbo-loading is, I have to put an end to the good news and tell you to stay away from snacks and fatty foods. This is a bummer, but I'm sure the carbs will help ease the pain. Also, please note that you cannot carbo-load in one day; it takes several days for your body to store up the glycogen (carb-related energy stuff) it will need on race day. So, start this utopia of carbs and rest at least three days before you go off to the anti-utopia that is a marathon.

The day before the marathon, continue taking in as much water and carbs as you can stand and try to avoid salty foods and protein (pork rinds are totally out). I highly recommend sticking with food you know your stomach likes. This is not the time to have your digestive tract go on strike. Another way to avoid stomach issues during the race is to avoid salad and vegetables the day before your event (seriously, best diet ever).

Although you'll be looking for something to do during your week of nonmovement, that nonmovement shouldn't include a sports massage, unfortunately. I know a massage should never be wrong; but if you've had a sports massage you'll understand that there is very little right about the strain these things put on your poor helpless muscles. In the weeks before a marathon, a sports massage can bully your muscles into working better, but the week before a marathon, you're trying to rest your muscles, not torture them anymore. So stay away from the sports massage.

As hard as it is to believe, you'll actually be doing something other than just scarfing down carbs and resting this week. You'll also be planning your Marathon Outfit. The general rule for this, just like other aspects of preparation, is to stick with what you know. Your shorts, shoes, and sports bra have had months to adapt to you and you to them. Do not bring visitors into the mix now. Your body will not welcome them. If you train with a group, you might receive a team singlet (shirt) to wear on marathon day. This is a great way to spot your team members among the thousands of runners, but it's also a great source of chafing if you aren't careful. Make sure to wash the singlet when you get it and then take it out for at least one run before the marathon. This will give you an idea of how it rubs and where to apply BODYGLIDE to avoid raw armpits. Raw armpits can be a bit of a downer.

If you are traveling by plane to your marathon, it's wise to take all your major marathon clothes in your carry-on. No one wants to see your naked butt running barefoot on the marathon course because the airline lost your luggage, and you can't wear anything new on marathon day. Even if you're not traveling out of town, it may feel that way because of all the crap you have to get together to take with you to the race. (See Appendix B, "Your Marathon Checklist," on page 227, for a full listing of crap.) You will probably take a look at your pile of race-day necessities and wonder whether it would hurt your time to pull a suitcase behind you during the run. If you can fit a lounge chair into that suitcase, I say go for it.

WHAT TO EXPECT ON THE DAY OF THE MARATHON

Oh my god, marathon day. Try not to hyperventilate.

Continue your now-legendary water intake until about fifteen minutes before the race starts. Try to use the restroom before you take off; the bathroom situation along the route can be a bit sketchy. Prepare yourself for more behind-a-tree accommodations and fewer available port-a-potties. To reduce your odds of getting arrested for public urination, use the bathroom before you start your race.

In addition to drinking water, eat a small snack before your run. Make sure this is something you've tested out before other long runs so you know that it won't leave you huddled in a ball on the side of the course at Mile 4.

Now you're totally enriched and are ready to go. While you wait for the race to start, make sure you stop and take in the whole pre-marathon buzz. People are pumped, they're anxious, and they are all going to look like walking piles of crap the next time you see them at the end of the race. So appreciate the beauty while you can. Also appreciate that you are standing at the start line of a friggin' marathon. Absorb that fact for a moment and remind yourself exactly how much ass you kick for seeing your training all the way through to this start line. No matter what happens for the next twenty-six miles, you've accomplished a great thing the past few months. Just by standing there you've far exceeded your preconceived notions of what you could do. Now, in the next twenty-six miles, get ready to exceed even more.

Go ahead and take a picture. The "before" photos are always charming, with all their hope and innocence.

Once you're off on the marathon route, you should be pretty well trained in how to handle yourself. Stay hydrated; drink the water and sports drinks offered at aid stations. Try to maintain the pace and strategy you've built over the last few months; focus on knocking off a mile at a time, instead of worrying about the distance ahead. There's probably no way to do this, but I thought I'd throw it out there in hopes you have mental capabilities greater than mine. Trust me, that shouldn't be much of a challenge.

POST-MARATHON

If your post-marathon does not include a visit to the hospital, consider the event a smashing success. But then again, I'm easily impressed when it comes to running abilities.

After you've completed your marathon, you'll have yet another set of overwhelming emotions running through you, ranging from elation to exhaustion to letdown. It will be easy to be swept up by these emotions for a while. Regardless of whether you hit a high or a low, keep a few details in mind.

Try not to sit down (or collapse) immediately following your race. Doing so might cause your muscles to tighten up to the point where you'll feel like you can never stand up again. Try to keep moving and maybe stretch a little.

It is very important to continue drinking fluids. Your body is thirsty, and hungry for that matter, so find something carb-tastic to replenish your empty reserves. I know that eating and drinking after a marathon might not seem like the most appealing thing in the world, but doing so will keep you healthy and feeling better the next day. Most marathons offer various foods and drinks at the finish line. You can kill all sorts of birds with one stone if you wander around food tables, eating and drinking and not collapsing on the ground. You are such a multitasker!

Go ahead and take a picture. The "after" photos are quite charming as well. It's not every day you get a photo of yourself that looks like you've been run over by a bulldozer while wearing spandex.

After you get back home or to the hotel, continue to eat, but this time a nice balanced meal. I tell you this because that's what a book should tell you, but I will also tell you that I went back and had room service bring me the biggest hamburger and order of french fries ever known to mankind. Balanced shmalanced. I'd never been this hungry in my life, and if some friggin' nutritionists thought I was going to waste this hunger on a balanced meal, then they were as high as I wish I'd been at Mile 15.

As far as the rest of the day goes, it's recommended you keep the carbs coming at dinner, because your body will still be needing the wonders that only carbs can provide. You burned about 8,000 calories, so go ahead and eat up. You so earned it. The rest of the night is up to you and how you are feeling. You might be on an excitement high or an exhaustion low. Regardless, try to celebrate your accomplishment at least a little bit. If you're up for it, join your fellow runners at a post-marathon get-together where you can celebrate and rehash your marathon glory. Plus, you all will look hilarious as you limp along together, your faces covered in grimaces, the least intimidating street gang ever. (Unless of course you're near an all-you-can-eat-buffet restaurant. In which case you will be one of the most intimidating, aggressive groups ever seen.)

No matter how your marathon turned out, no matter how great your time was, no matter how many times you cried while you were running (it happens to the best of us), do not ever let yourself feel anything besides pride for finishing not only the race but the months of training that led you there. When you started this running insanity it was heavy on insanity and light on running; but by the end, the scales seem to balance a bit. You have taken on a seemingly impossible task and have not only done it, but have proven that "impossible" is just a state of mind. When you cross the finish line of your marathon you will, in effect, be crossing a huge goal off your list. No matter how you got to that finish line, no matter how many ups and downs marked your route, you will forever be a Marathoner. And that's pretty damn cool. Now go have your way with that all-you-can-eat buffet to celebrate.

●●●

Journal Entry: WEEK 16
The End of the Road

So where do I start in recapping my Hawaiian marathon? How do I adequately relate the glory of every single heel-to-toe step I took? This could be a really long journal entry, 'cause I took *a lot* of steps. We'll do the math on how many steps I took a little later in the broadcast. But first, I'd like to clear up a slight misconception and a very large lack of faith on the part of my friends and family. A day or two after My Marathon, I emailed everyone and stated that the good news was that I did okay for thirteen miles. Then I stated that the bad news was that a marathon is twenty-six miles. Many of my friends and family of little faith thought those statements meant I stopped the marathon after thirteen miles. Apparently they thought my slogan was, "When the going gets tough, the tough go sit on a beach instead of finishing what they've been training months for, and raised four grand for." I had several emails and voice messages when I returned from Hawaii reassuring me that it was quite alright that I didn't finish and I should still be proud of myself. *What the?* How could these people possibly think I wasn't going to finish that marathon?

I had run hundreds of miles in preparation for this marathon, I had a goal, I had a dream, I was everywoman; but mostly I had quite a few people who had donated money. There was no way I was going to tell them I quit at Mile 13. What if they wanted their money back? And more important, what if they still expected me to run a marathon? I couldn't fathom starting another one of these things, so I just finished the one I was already doing. With not one damn taxicab anywhere along the marathon route, I didn't have much

>>>

>>>

choice but to keep moving. And moving, and moving, and then moving some more.

The moving started at about 3 AM when Chipper Jen woke me up with her chipper nature that apparently needs no sleep to thrive. Thank god I'm hard of hearing. I didn't put my hearing aids in for at least a half hour. I couldn't deal with the impending marathon, the fact that it was 3 AM, *and* Jen's positive attitude all at the same time. A girl can only take so much.

We made our way down to the lobby of the hotel so that we could meet with the rest of our team. These people were apparently told that it was Christmas morning, Elvis was performing, and someone was handing out free pie all at the same time, because that's how excited they were. They obviously didn't know we were about to start a marathon. I let them continue on in their delusional state and I stayed strong as the only person who really knew what was going on here.

Once we started our walk to the start line, I was struck by a number of things that just didn't seem right. The first and most obvious of these things had to be the fact that we were *walking* to the start line, which was a mile from our hotel. Someone actually said, "Well what's another mile? I mean, we're already running twenty-six, might as well go for twenty-seven." We didn't even get to credit that mile toward our 26.2. What kind of injustice is that? Some people were jogging that mile. I was gonna join them, but then I decided to just jab myself in the eye with a stick because that made just about as much sense.

I was also a little worried when my right knee began to hurt during the walk to the start line. That's

>>>

>>>

always a good sign, right? Yes, things can only turn out well when you are in pain before the marathon even starts.

Then I noticed that I was wearing a tank top and spandex shorts. Now normally the horrendous visual of this combination would worry me on its own. But I wasn't as worried about fashion as I was about the time of day and the fact that I was already warm. You see, it was about 3:45 AM, pitch dark, and the middle of December. And I wasn't even remotely cold wearing only a tank top and shorts. I realized things might not turn out so well when the sun came up and brought its trademark heating mechanisms with it.

Despite these early signs of marathon trouble ahead, I continued on to the start line. I don't think I had much choice really. There were about 25,000 people getting ready to run. Not to mention 80,000 spectators (almost all of them Japanese and assorted Americans) who thought it would be good times to get up at 4 AM just to watch people run away from them. I was caught up in this mob of run-happy people, and for my own well-being I just continued on in the direction they were heading.

Because there were so many runners, we were only able to get within a half mile of the start line. We crowded around, waiting for Christmas or Elvis or the pie to show up. This was good because my knee appreciated the rest. During this time I fully assembled myself. In addition to my already-stylish outfit, I added my water-bottle holder around my waist. I then safety-pinned baggies full of inspirational quotes and bananas (separate baggies) to my waist. Then I tied a bandana around my water-bottle holder, just in case I needed to put ice in it later. There was also the off

>>>

>>>

chance that I was going to have to put my kneecap in it when it fell off later. Although it was against the rules, I clipped my radio on my belt and put my headphones on. Apparently runners aren't supposed to wear head-phones during the race, because not hearing might cause them to run into someone or miss hearing the combination of Japanese rally cries and the runners' shrieks of pain throughout the race. And you really wouldn't want to miss all that. Unfortunately, I can't hear very well even if I'm not wearing headphones, so my chances of running into someone weren't going to be affected by the headphones. And my chances of running twenty-six miles without some sort of music were about as good as my chances of being one of the people speaking Japanese. So I put the headphones on and dared someone to tell me to take them off.

For fueling purposes, I safety-pinned three GU pack-ets to my shirt. I also attached my runner number. The runner number would identify me in case the three GU packets proved ineffective and I ended up passing out and having to be carried to the nearest hospital or beachfront bar with umbrella drinks.

Now that I was fully assembled, I was ready for this race to start. I was pumped, I was psyched, I was really wanting to puke or go back to bed. Shortly before the race started, fireworks exploded and someone sang the national anthem and the crowd cheered and I'm pretty sure Whitney Houston was there singing "One Moment in Time." Or that might have just been my imagination. There's no way Whitney Houston would have been up at 5 AM.

Then someone shot the start gun and we were *off!* Well, we weren't really *off!* so much as we were *be-ing slowly removed!* Because of the mob of runners, it

>>>

>>>

took us about fifteen minutes just to get to the start line, after the race had started. This was a great fifteen minutes for me, the only time when Jen and I were running at the same pace, a great pace, a pace I would revisit later in the marathon.

The first couple of miles went pretty quickly, because I was running with 25,000 people. I had no idea where I was or how far I had gone. I didn't know where the mile marker signs were supposed to be, so I couldn't figure out how far along I was. The only signs I saw were ones that said how many *K*'s I had gone. Seriously, can we not come together as a world and figure out one way (our way) to measure distances? They might as well have had a sign that read "3 PQYU" for all the significance "3 K" had to me. (Thinking about it now, I was probably way too concerned about finding out how far I'd gone when I was still within the first five miles. But it seemed important to me at the time.)

My coaches had instructed me to take the first thirteen miles slow to increase the chances of me actually seeing the second thirteen miles. I was also trying to stop at every mile marker to stretch and walk a little. This made for a ridiculously slow pace, but at least I was running. And I wasn't crying. Yet.

At Mile 5, a mean-spirited assface (I apologize for the language, but you will soon see that it is completely justified and pretty much the only word on the planet to describe this person) decided it would be fun to hold a sign that read YOU'RE ALMOST THERE! Yeah, if I was almost there then he was almost not an assface.

At Mile 6, a tragedy of epic proportions struck. No, Chipper Jen didn't stop smiling while bopping along. There's no way I could have gone on after something

>>>

like that occurred. Not that I would have known what Jen was doing; she was all the way to Mile 12 by that point. No, the tragedy struck as I went through one of the aid stations set up along the route. I grabbed two cups of water, one to drink and one to pour on my head. I was hoping that by keeping myself fully drenched I would avoid death by heat exhaustion. This would give dehydration, malnutrition, cramping, and extreme pain a better chance of being the cause of my demise.

The complexity of walking, drinking, and pouring all at the same time left no brain power to remember to remove my headphones before I poured water on my head. Future reference: Water and tiny Walkmans don't really mix well. Now don't worry, the head-phones didn't stop working. No, no, no, they kept working perfectly. Despite the itty-bitty fact that they were now stuck on one station. Oh yeah. With twenty miles to go, I was stuck on an R&B/hip-hop station. That may not seem that bad, right? Well, it was "Milkshake" Weekend on this station, which meant the song "Milkshake" was playing every other minute. For those who don't know "Milkshake," consider yourselves very, very, very lucky. Do not seek it out, do not ask anyone about it, just go on about your lives and be thankful that you've never heard these lines repeated at least forty-five times in the course of a three-minute song:

My Milkshake brings all the boys to the yard,
And their like "It's better than yours"
Damn right, It's better than yours,
I can teach you, but I have to charge

(I actually went to Lyrics.com to look up those lyrics because I thought I had them wrong. Because they

>>>

make no sense whatsoever. But then again the video for this song features a bunch of girls in a diner throwing milkshakes all over themselves while wearing very tight shorts and tank tops. Let's just say I don't think they're wearing those outfits to prepare for a marathon.) I'm sure there are many fans of this song out there, and I don't mean to offend their (horrible) taste in music. It's just that while you run, music is pretty much the only thing that can get your mind off the fact that you have not only subjected yourself, of your own free will, to the worst pain of your life, but you've decided to go ahead and pick an event in which the pain can last for the better part of a workday.

My Milkshake brings all the boys to the yard,
And their like "It's better than yours"
Damn right, It's better than yours,
I can teach you, but I have to charge

This song replaying over and over was not helping me through my pain. At all.

At Mile 7, I cemented the fact that I'm not at all a Serious Runner (not that I didn't know this before). As I mentioned earlier, I had decided to pin a baggie of bananas to my belt. I had cut up two bananas and put them in a baggie honestly thinking that they would stay in banana form for twenty-six miles. The pinning of the bananas hadn't gone quite as well as planned, so I had to resort to stuffing the bag in a small little zippered pouch on my belt thingy. Well, as you can probably imagine, the stuffing of bananas is not conducive to keeping them in non-mush form. So when I went to get the bananas out of my pouch at Mile 7, it turned out that I had succeeded in making my very own GU-like product. Quite exciting, and my first entrepreneurial effort as well. The contents of

>>>

>>>

the baggie weren't visually appealing but they were still bananas, so I decided to squeeze some banana GU into my mouth, zip the baggie up, stuff it back in my pouch, and be on my newly enriched way.

This plan seemed to work fine until shortly after Mile 7, when I felt something very questionable splatter against my leg. A large portion of my Banana GU was sliding down my leg and another portion had splattered on the ground behind me. Oh, did I mention that the zippered pouch was on my back? Yeah, it was. Oh, did I mention that it was still kind of dark along the route? Yeah, it was. Did I mention how many disgusted people were running behind me wondering what exactly was falling from my backside? Yeah, there were quite a few.

Around Miles 8 and 9, the knee started hurting pretty good, but I kept going because the sooner I finished, the sooner I would stop hearing "Milkshake."

At Mile 10, I took my headphones off to avoid listening to 50 Cent rap about being shot again. As soon as I took them off, I was bombarded with people screaming, "Go AIDS!" "Go leukemia!" "Go short-term memory!" "Go diabetes!" "Go stroke!" "Go short-term memory!" I might be making up the short-term memory one, but the rest I actually heard. It turns out that quite a few runners were doing the marathon as a fundraiser for the various diseases and afflictions of the world. And there were hundreds of people on the sidelines cheering us on. The combination of yelling supporters and sweating runners was at once bizarre, touching, and thought-provoking. It's pretty awesome that so many runners were running for something greater than themselves and raising money for so many good causes. And it was pretty cool that people

>>>

>>>

were willing to stand on the sidelines for hours holding signs and cheering in the hopes of helping even one runner through another mile. But was all this really necessary? There has got to be an alternative form of fundraising. Those Girl Scouts have the right idea with that whole Thin Mint thing. They raise millions of dollars with those cookies. And those cookies are something worth cheering about.

Between Miles 10 and 13 things got a little blurry. Several things most likely happened during those miles, but I'm a little hazy on specifics. I know my knee started hurting pretty bad within those miles. I started pulling my inspirational quotes out of my baggie with vigor in an attempt to divert my attention away from the pain. Remember how I'd asked for funny quotes to make me smile? Yeah, they weren't working. I wasn't smiling.

Somewhere around these miles, we came to a hill with an incline of approximately 93 degrees. It went on for at least ten miles. I'm sure of it. Another lovely feature of this hill was that it was the same hill the runners ran down on their way to the finish line. This meant that around my Mile 12 I was watching runners coming at me who were at their Mile 20. This was not good for my mental state.

Seriously, I think my biggest problem was the mental thing. I could not take it one mile at a time. I just kept thinking of how many miles I had to go and that depressed me and made my knee hurt even more. Seeing these happy-ass runners at Mile 20 when I was only at Mile 12 only reminded me of how far I had to go and how many other people were already where I had to go. It was the equivalent of being kicked on my way down.

>>>

>>>

Shortly before the Mile 13 marker, I decided I needed to walk for a while. My knee was hurting like hell and the rest of my body wasn't feeling much better. It was then, at the start of what was to be the longest thirteen miles of my life, that I saw a very excited Chipper Jen running toward me, down the hill I was walking up. She waved vigorously and smiled brightly. I frowned and might have raised my eyebrows slightly as a sign of recognition, but I am not sure I even had the motivation to exert that much effort.

At the next aid station I saw a bunch of people kneeling on piles of bagged ice. I think the ice was meant for the cups of water being handed out, but the runners thought it would be better put to use on their aching knees. I buried my knee in one bag and hoped it would numb the pain. It seemed to work, but the main problem was the fact that I couldn't duct-tape the bag of ice to my knee to keep it numb for the rest of the marathon.

When I started walking again, it became obvious that I was going to be walking for the remainder of the marathon. I began to experience stabbing pains on the outside and inside of my knee, not to mention the pain shooting down from my knee to my foot with every step. I just don't know if I can adequately explain how great this all felt. And knowing I still had thirteen miles to go . . . it was just lovely.

I walked another mile or two and began to realize the consequences of training to run a marathon and instead *walking* it. It turns out that running and walking use very different muscles in my already-malfunctioning legs. These muscles began to express their disinterest in the marathon around this time. Most notably the muscles behind my knees were on fire. You'd think those

>>>

>>>

muscles would have had a little workout during the 275 miles I had run since August. Guess not. My feet were also shooting pains up to meet the ones that were coming down from my knees. In all the time I had run, my feet had never hurt before. As good a day as any to start, I guess.

In a bizarre twist of irony, I began walking like my grandfather used to walk. After his stroke, he lost some use of his body, which caused him to drag one of his legs slightly as he walked. Here I was raising funds for the American Stroke Association, dragging my un-bendable leg along for thirteen miles. It was almost poetic. Not quite as poetic as "My Milkshake brings all the boys to the yard," but close.

Just past the next aid station I finally succumbed to the urge that had been building up inside of me for the past few miles to cry like a baby. I'd been fighting back tears with every step and figured maybe it would take less energy to just get the crying over with. I sat on the curb next to the ice bags and covered my face while I cried. Midway through my cry, a woman kneeled in the ice next to me and said, "I wish I could somehow cover my entire body with this ice." I of-fered to cover her in ice if she would lay down on the ground, but we agreed that it probably wouldn't help too much.

I left her kneeling on the ice and began dragging myself along again. As I hobbled along I noticed other people hobbling around me. I've never seen a more pathetic group. We looked like the Land of the Walking Dead. Some people were crying; others were passed out on the ground; others limped as if they'd just been shot. We looked like extras for a cheesy

>>>

>>>

zombie or war movie. We were the zombies and we were definitely post-battle.

Later, a girl in front of me unknowingly dropped her hair scrunchie on the ground. Two girls walking near me also noticed it. We knew that the nice human thing to do would be to pick it up and give it back to the girl who dropped it. But as we looked from the scrunchie to the scrunchie girl, none of us could possibly imagine ever again moving fast enough to catch up with the scrunchie owner. We stared at the scrunchie for what seemed like forever. Much to the relief of the other two I finally said, "I'll get it." They gave me a slight smile then hobbled away. I managed to pick it up and did my best interpretation of rapid movement in an effort to get to the scrunchie owner. When I finally caught up to her she merely gave me a "Thanks," then zoomed off at her sixteen-minute-mile pace. Normally, I would have gotten angry, but instead I just cried some more.

At about Mile 20 I had been running/walking/crying for about five and a half hours. A runner from our stroke team came up behind me and asked how I was doing. I said not so great. He said that he was surprised he had made it to Mile 20 because he had broken a rib and sprained both his feet recently. Such joy it brought me that the man with broken ribs and no feet had caught up to me.

He told me he took some ibuprofen a few miles back, which really helped. "What?!" I very calmly asked. You see, we had been very clearly warned not to take ibuprofen while running the marathon because of what it does to your liver or something. But the man with no ribs said that's just a precaution; and unless you've been a raging alcoholic for twenty years, your liver

>>>

>>>

should be able to handle ibuprofen without exploding or doing whatever livers do when they malfunction.

I couldn't believe this. I wanted to take drugs so bad but hadn't because of the whole liver explosion thing. Now this man with no ribs or feet was passing me because of all the drugs he took. I was so jealous. I was going to continue walking with him, but I had to sit down at every mile marker and pull my leg up to my chest for a while. Therefore the footless, drugged man continued on without me.

At Mile 21, I began losing any sense of humor I might have had left. I wanted drugs and I wanted them now. Instead of safety-pinning any more inspirational quotes to my shirt, I started taking them off. They, along with everything in my sight, annoyed me. I was pissed off, I was hot, I was in pain, and I was sure Chipper Jen was already back at the hotel with an umbrella drink.

At this point, I passed a woman on the sidelines who was dressed in American flag-patterned clothes and was playing the accordion while her dog sat next to her listening. I have no idea what this lady was doing or why she was doing it, but she was responsible for the one single smile I cracked during my entire twenty-six miles. The combination of her accordion and my delirium made me laugh for approximately twenty-four seconds. Then I was pissed again.

Some American Stroke Association team people were at Mile 22. I could tell by the way they looked at me that I looked as horrible as I felt. They ran up and asked if I needed anything. I didn't want to speak to them too much, because if they'd asked how I was doing, I would have curled up in a ball and cried

>>>

>>>

for three days straight. I told them I wanted drugs, now. While one rooted through her bag in search of drugs, the other asked earnestly if she could get me anything else. I very politely said, "A new &*^$%** knee." "Well, um, we don't have one of those. How 'bout some Wheat Thins?" "Fine." I took the drugs and Wheat Thins and some water and continued on with my &*^$%** knee.

A half mile later one of our coaches came running up to me with an expression on her face that looked as if she's just found out that Bambi died. From a reasonable distance, she asked if I had everything I needed. I nodded yes, trying hard not to burst into tears. I found out later that shortly after an eighty-year-old couple crossed the finish line, Jen had emergency personnel radio our coach to tell her she was worried and to keep an eye out for me. Hence the Bambi look.

Around Mile 24, my drugs kicked in and my knee began feeling better. Now all I had to deal with was my aching muscles and bad attitude. Since I'd walked so long at such a slow pace I wasn't that tired and I was able to start power walking. Everyone around me in the Land of the Walking Dead was barely moving. By comparison I was Speedy Gonzales, blazing past everyone with the new energy and excitement provided by the drugs and by the fact that I was almost done. I almost felt guilty ditching all the people who'd staggered along with me the past ten miles. Almost.

When I hit Mile 25 I decided my knee was cured and I would run the last mile because, oh my god, if she brings her Milkshake to the yard one more time. . . .

As I began to run it became quite obvious that the ibuprofen had not cured my knee. But I didn't care, I was

>>>

>>>

running, I was getting to the finish, and I was gonna try my hardest not to cry. I looked up to see the sign 1 K UNTIL THE FINISH. What?! What is 1 K? A little help for the nonmetric people please! How far is 1 friggin' K?! I saw a corner up ahead and I was convinced that the finish line would be located a mere yard and a half beyond that. Much to my dismay, it was an aid station. I don't want an aid station! I want the finish line! Keep your sports drink and your sponges and your ice. I just want the finish line.

In the middle of this internal rant, I spotted the finish line, still approximately two time zones away. But at least I had visual confirmation of its existence. I tried to run faster toward the big FINISH sign, but I swear it kept moving away from me. It was like those horror movies when the camera zooms in on a person but the background keeps receding. It was horrifying.

Finally I reached the finish. Just behind a seven-year-old kid with crutches. As it turns out, my actual slogan is something closer to "When the going gets tough, the tough sit down and cry, then get back up and limp to the finish, but not before stopping to cry a few more times." It's quite catchy. I think I'll have it printed up on T-shirts and hats and whatnot.

After I crossed the finish line, Chipper Jen and I promptly went back to the hotel, ordered quite a bit of room service, and sprawled out on our respective beds eating said room service. We covered our aching bodies in ice and Aspercreme in hopes of ceasing the throbbing pains. My aches weren't really alleviated, but I can't tell you how excited I was that Jen was finally in some pain. She finally understood what I went through after every run, whether it was one mile or twenty-six. "Oh my god that hurts," she kept saying

>>>

>>>

about her knees. It took twenty-six miles and many months, but Jen finally had a friggin' leg cramp. Ah, it's the little things in life. . . .

In the days following our marathon we were quite sore, but we were also in Hawaii, something I was oblivious to until the moment I finished the marathon. I'm happy to report that we drank many tropical beverages and actually made special requests for umbrellas in pretty much every drink we ordered, even water. Because even water deserves to be festive, you know.

So here we are at the conclusion of my Marathon Madness. It's the end of an era really. A short era, yes, but an era nonetheless. How can I sum up the past months? "Ouch" might be adequate, but I feel this experience deserves something more.

When I asked my fellow marathoners why they were doing this awful, awful activity, many stated that it was something on their list of things to do before they died. You know those lists Oprah encourages that often involve skydiving or seeing all Seven Wonders or, in my case, setting the all-time record for the most consecutive hours spent watching DVDs. Everyone has dreams.

But I never had a marathon on any list of anything I ever even wanted to watch other people do. So what was I doing at that marathon, and why had I devoted months to training for it? Like many things you do in life, there wasn't just one reason. It started because my grandfather had passed away and I wanted to do something, anything, to honor his memory. When the marathon postcard arrived in the mail, I thought maybe this was what I was supposed to do. I also

>>>

>>>

thought my grandpa would have been just as proud if I'd sold Thin Mints. But the Girl Scouts never sent a postcard. Dammit.

Then I went to the marathon information meeting and thought it over for a few weeks before I even mentioned it to anyone. I've never been one to stick around when things get tough or I start feeling a little defeated. In the figurative sense, I've been a runner my whole life. How ironic that running became the first difficult thing that I couldn't run away from? Oh how the mind boggles.

Why the first thing I decided to finish was friggin' twenty-six miles long I have no idea. I couldn't have started with a fifty-yard dash? Geez. But no matter how ridiculous the goal, I kept putting on those shoes and that spandex and those headphones. I kept running. The perfectionist who never likes to play unless she can win kept playing even though she obviously wasn't going to win anything. Unless it was the award for the most creative combination of cuss words assembled while kicking a drinking fountain.

I found inspiration in the tiniest and largest of places. There was the little poodle dog I nicknamed Cujo that repeatedly tried to attack me during my eighteen-mile run, providing me with much-needed humor and something to run away from. There were the people who donated money to a great cause but also to the fact that they thought I could do this. There was the limping man during the marathon who so needed a cup of water but instead offered it to another runner who looked like she needed it more. There was the postcard my friend put in my bag to surprise me when I got to Hawaii that read simply, "I'm proud of you." There were the countless emails from friends

>>>

>>>

and family that said I was doing a good thing and/or I was a complete moron. There were the people who showed up and washed cars for hours to help us raise money. There was the lady at Mile 23 who had a sign taped to her back that read, PLEASE GOD, LET THERE BE SOMEONE BEHIND ME TO READ THIS. There was my grandfather and others like him who would have given anything to be able to complain about running twenty-six miles. There was Chipper Jen, always waiting for me, sometimes for hours, at the finish line. And, of course, there were pineapple drinks.

All these things and many others ran through my head during the 275 miles I ran over the course of my training, or the 28,800 steps I took during the marathon (I did the math based on an average of one step per second). They all got me to the finish line. With a little help from the Banana GU.

Am I hoping my marathon inspires others to lace up their running shoes and aim for next year's Honolulu Marathon? I'm not sure. I will tell aspiring marathoners they can do it. No matter who they are, they can do it. So, they can't use that as a reason not to start running. They are, however, more than welcome to use chafing and spandex as reasons to not run.

Even though I can't tell others whether they should chase their marathon dreams, I highly recommend they do something completely out of character, something they never in a million years thought they'd do, something they may fail miserably at. Because sometimes the places where you end up finding your true self are the places you never thought to look.

That, and I don't want to be the only one who sucks at something.

>>>

>>>

Have I hung up my running shoes for good? I doubt it. I'm not ready to hang up the mass quantities of calories I can get away with eating while using those shoes. Now that I don't *have* to run, I might enjoy it— *might* being the operative word. And while I recognize that I accomplished something by getting to the finish line, I really don't feel like I accomplished everything I could have. So although it was never there in the first place, now on my list of things to do before I die is *Finish a marathon in under five hours.*

Yeah, I know I finished, but I know I could do better. Maybe not this year, maybe not next year, maybe not until someone offers me some Oprah type of money, and maybe not before technology can build me a new knee. But someday I'll do it again. For now I'm gonna get back to setting that DVD-watching record. Baby steps.

My Marathon brings my body to tears,
And I'm like "This is insane,"
Damn right, this is insane,
I can stop, but I can't find a cab.

Epilogue

So here we are at the end of your marathon journey. And what a journey it's been. I always joke that when you train for a marathon, you're really just running in a series of circles because you always end up right where you started, no matter how many damn miles you ran. Yet after my marathon, I realized that although I was geographically in the same place in which I'd begun, I wasn't anywhere near where I had started as a person. The changes were obvious, but not necessarily to the naked eye. Sure, my body had changed: It had become toned where it had once been loose; it had become damaged where it had once been pristine from years of nonmovement; it had become tough where it had once been a little wimpy. But more than any exterior changes, I noticed changes within. I was starting to become the kind of person I'd always wanted to be.

It's all very Oprah "Live Your Best Life" of me, but I now see that my marathon marked a very real shift between being a person who talks about things and a person who does things. My training wasn't so much about the running as it was about the challenge and how I approached it. It turned out to be the first in a series of challenges I took on. Because, honestly, after you drag your leg for thirteen miles in the scorching sun while listening to "Milkshake" for hours on end, you start to think you can take on pretty much anything (as long is it doesn't involve hip-hop music).

The specific challenges I took on following my marathon aren't really important; what is important is for you to do the same. Recognize what you've done in completing this tremendously difficult task and the inner resources you used to accomplish it. You'll be able to tap those same resources to accomplish other things in your life. (Advil can help other dreams come true, right?)

Also recognize that although your body is unhappy with you right now, and is demanding some mandatory recliner time as a result, you finished a damn marathon and are alive to tell the tale. The fact that you didn't perish either while training or running the actual marathon means that your body is up for a challenge now and then. I'm not saying it's gonna be happy about it, but once in a while it's important to see exactly how pissed off you can make your muscles. Some people call this masochism; I call it personal growth. (But that might be because I have developed quite an affinity for Advil.)

Do yourself a favor and review the journal entries and lists you've jotted down while taking on this challenge. You will see that the journey has involved more than just running; you've explored and found ways to take your body and mind out of your comfort zone and into a foreign (and very uncomfortable) land. The resources you used to navigate that land are the same ones you can use to navigate anything else that comes your way. Except don't wait for the challenges to come your way. Go looking for them. And when you do. I guarantee you'll find even more of yourself waiting there for you.

Well done, soldier, well done.

APPENDIX *A*
Your Accessory Checklist

Here is a handy list to take with you as you brave the world of running stores.

CLOTHES
❑ **Shoes**

Yes, I know you want the cutest ones, but get the ones that are the best fit, even if they don't have the exact color combination you want.

❑ **Running Shorts**

Say it with me now: "I will not purchase short shorts. I do not care if other super-fast Serious Runners wear them. I care about the well-being of my fellow runners and my un-tanned butt."

❑ **Sports Bra**

Choose wisely, the girls are countin' on ya.

❑ **Socks**

Cotton is rotten. And double lining is awesome. (Hey, give me a break, you try to find something that rhymes with "rotten.")

❑ **Shirts**

Here's where you can choose primarily on cuteness. Go ahead, get flashy. You know you want to.

❑ **Hat**

Don't worry, everyone will be wearing the weird hat with all the holes in it, so you won't look that strange.

STUFF
❑ **Walkman or iPod**

Get a Walkman or an iPod, or simply be left with your own thoughts during your runs. Take my word for it, you really don't have nearly as many thoughts as you think you have.

❏ **Water-Holder Butt Thingy**
You probably don't want to call it this when inquiring about it at the local running store. I don't want you to look like a fool. You'll have plenty of time for that after you actually put the Water-Holder Butt Thingy on.

❏ **Watch**
It's fun to see how your time improves . . . if you don't throw the watch away during your frustrating first weeks.

❏ **Gatorade**
Do not be disappointed if you don't actually sweat cool colors after drinking this stuff. I know, I believed the commercials too.

❏ **GU**
Instead of buying a lot of one flavor right off the bat, buy one of each to decide which one you actually like and which one won't make you nauseated at Mile 18. Well, any more nauseated than you'll already be at Mile 18.

❏ **BODYGLIDE**
Go ahead and splurge for your own sake. You probably don't want to be asking your fellow runners if you can borrow theirs after they're done applying it down their pants.

THE MOST IMPORTANT STUFF
❏ **Journal**
Oprah will be so proud!

❏ **Camera—Still and Video**
Your ass will never look this good again, so take pictures. Lots of them.

❏ **People**
You'll need them for moral support and/or to carry you home.

APPENDIX *B*

Your Marathon Checklist

❑ **Running shoes and socks**
If you don't remember these, I'm thinking the rest of the list may be moot.

❑ **Running Outfit**
Try to look cute; there will be pictures.

❑ **Race number and safety pins**
Safety pins are very important, it's not going to be fun to try to hold that race number to your chest through the entire marathon.

❑ **Water to drink before**
Booze to drink after.

❑ **Clothes to wear over your Running Outfit if it's cold before the race**
They should probably be clothes you don't mind throwing off once the cold is replaced by heatstroke.

❑ **Sports drink**
Or pick them up at the aid tables along the way.

❑ **GU-type stuff**
Use some extra safety pins to pin them to your shirt; you won't care at Mile 18 that you look ridiculous.

❑ **Baggies**
I know it seems weird, but these things come in so damn handy. You never know when you might need a baggie to hold any of the following: ice, munchies, ID, your kneecap.

❑ **Toilet paper**
Probably not the whole roll.

❑ **Ibuprofen**
Drugs are never a bad idea.

❏ **Money**
For emergencies, like a cab or a beer.

❏ **BODYGLIDE**
A moped would probably help your body glide more, though.

❏ **A bag of clothes to change into after you're done**
Because you will be disgusting.

❏ **Post-marathon munchies**
Maybe an extra-large pizza, and then a main course, too.

APPENDIX *C*

Journal It

Look at you! Getting all introspective with the journal! I'm so proud. As you've probably figured out by now, I enjoy putting a thought on paper. I recommend it to all of you as well. There's no need to be as long-winded as I am, but try to capture as many details as you can. Marathon training, like anything amazing (and painful), will someday be a distant memory (unless you still have a limp like I do). This journal space will let you revisit your marathon journey whenever you need a reminder of what happened during those months you spent in an Advil- and sweat-induced haze.

As you train for a marathon, you are taking on major physical and mental challenges. Use these pages, or post your thoughts on a blog, to describe how you're overcoming those challenges, even if your efforts consist mostly of cussing and ice. Use these pages to tell your marathon story as it is happening. If you do, it will serve as a reminder of how much butt you kicked (and how much kicked your butt). Introspect away!

My Journal

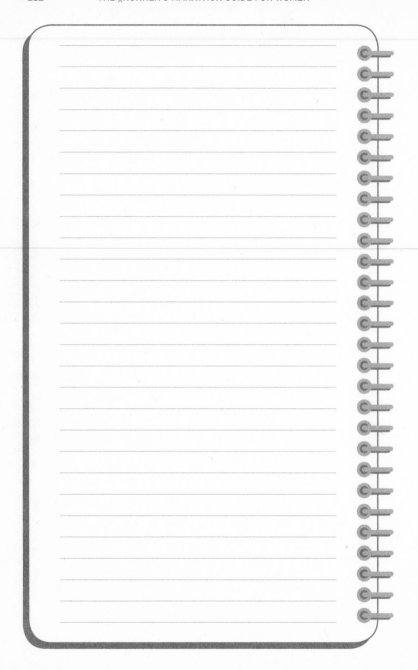

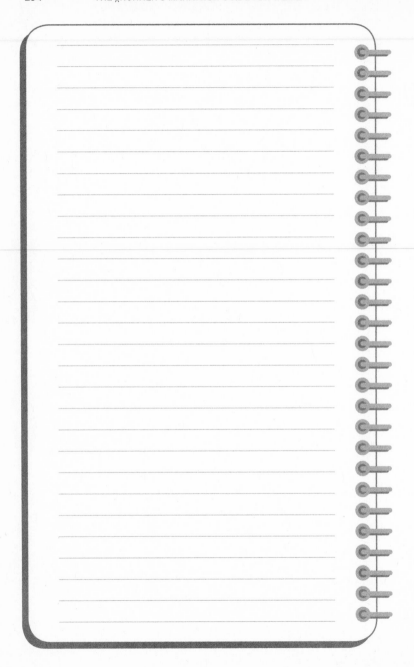

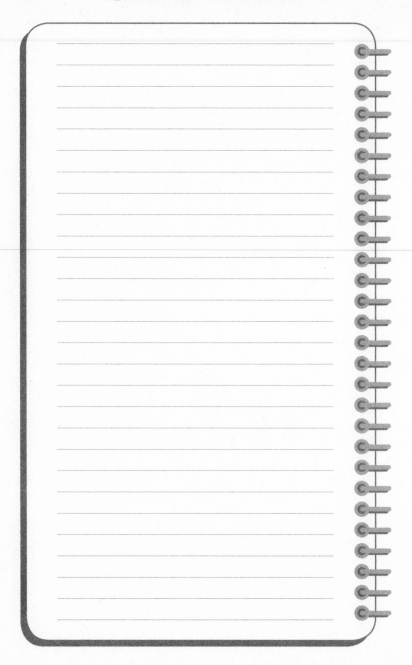

Resources

FUNDRAISING TRAINING TEAMS

Fundraising teams combine fundraising with marathon training, which sometimes seems like a lot to take on. But as you make your way through your difficult training, it's much easier to stick with the training if you are part of a group and have coaches and training seminars to push you along. Also, teams usually have really cool post-marathon parties, and who doesn't love a party?

Train to End Stroke

www.strokeassociation.org

This very program, sponsored by the American Stroke Association, got my ass across the finish line. If that ain't a roaring endorsement, I don't know what is. It offers full and half-marathon training and is sarcasm-friendly.

Leukemia & Lymphoma Society's Team in Training

www.teamintraining.org

These guys have all the bases covered. You can train to run or walk a whole marathon or half-marathon or participate in a triathlon or century (hundred-mile) bike ride. Basically if you are looking to sweat, this group has a way for you to raise money doing it.

National AIDS Marathon Training Program

www.aidsmarathon.com

You can train to run a full marathon or half-marathon with this six-month program.

Children's Tumor Foundation's NF Marathon Team

www.ctf.org/marathon

This team offers full marathon and half-marathon training.

Arthritis Foundation Joints in Motion

www.jointsinmotion.org

Not only can you train to run or walk a marathon, you can also train to take a hike on a challenging trail. This seems just random enough for me to explore further. I'll let you know how it goes.

Avon Walk for Breast Cancer

www.avonfoundation.org

This is a fundraising team for breast cancer that sponsors a two-day walk. The distance is self-determined, but the course allows you to "walk as far as you choose" (up to a marathon and a half). I don't know why it would take anyone two days to walk as far as they choose. That should only take like five minutes, or until you find the nearest ice cream shop, whichever comes first.

Susan G. Komen Breast Cancer Foundation 3-Day Walks

www.the3day.org

This team trains you to walk sixty miles over the course of three days. It doesn't sound nearly as much fun as that two-day one where you can stop whenever you feel like it.

LARGEST U.S. MARATHONS

1. ING New York City Marathon
2. LaSalle Bank Chicago Marathon
3. Honolulu Marathon
4. Los Angeles Marathon
5. Marine Corps Marathon (Washington, DC)
6. Boston Marathon
7. Coca-Cola Zero Rock 'n' Roll Marathon (San Diego, CA)
8. New Las Vegas Marathon
9. Twin Cities Marathon
10. Walt Disney World Marathon
11. P.F. Chang's Rock 'n' Roll Arizona Marathon (Phoenix, AZ)
12. Portland Marathon (OR)
13. Grandma's Marathon (Duluth, MN)
14. Citizen's Bank Philadelphia Marathon
15. Chevron Houston Marathon

Acknowledgments

To my agents, Lilly Ghahremani and Stefanie Von Borstel, for seeing something in me and my marathon tale, and working their butts off to make sure other people got to see it too. To my editor, Brooke Warner, whose helpful notes ("I just don't get this . . .") and even helpfuller editing of my sometimes horrendous misuse of the English language made me a better writer (who still doesn't know, when to use, commas).

To Bryan and Sheila DeBlonk, for letting me chase my dreams, while still keeping a job. To my peeps at CHA, most notably my ladies in the accounting department, for their support and their steady supply of cake and other celebratory snacks. My marathon training was the only time I didn't gain weight while working there.

To Lori May, Jeff Oberlatz, Michelle Mussuto, Ed Castro, Michelle Ward, and the rest of the American Stroke Association team for putting up with my incessant mocking of their positive nature.

To all of my Habitat for Humanity friends, for throwing starfish.

To Jodi Holmes and Sommer Wilson, my roommates during my training and during the writing of this book. It's not easy living with an insane person, and they both handled it brilliantly.

To Rachel Wanner, Heather Webster, Colleen Scotten, Todd Lampe, Mo Mata, Matt Kuiper, Kevin Miles, Tom Roche,

Vince Jacob, Lisa Rosati, Michaela Borris, Jason Auerbach, Jay Wester, Melanie Shanley, Peter Krysinski, Todd Heinrich, Rafeal Siegel, Nick Lee, Travis Henderson, and everyone else who made the race a hell of a lot more fun.

To Rose Marie Garofalo, for being both my friend and my family. To Katy Sparkman, who I have watched grow from a little kid into one of the coolest people I know.

To (Chipper) Jen Burrows, whose strength in marathon training and in life astounds me. The journey is all about who you travel with, and I couldn't have asked for a better (or a more ridiculously positive) sidekick.

To my mother, Betty Lou Dais, whose laughter taught me how to be funny and whose heart taught me who I wanted to be. To my father, Dave Dais, who played sports with me for hours at a time, teaching me to always play, always try, and always kick a little ass along the way.

Thank you.

About the Author

Dawn Dais has spent the better part of her life avoiding running, runners, and all things calorie-burning. When she is not taking on ridiculous physical challenges, such as finishing a marathon, she stays mostly stationary as a freelance writer and designer. Dais contributes to a number of local and national publications and has been featured on the well-known Quotable Cards series. Never say never—Dais continues to run, albeit very slowly. She lives in Sacramento, California.

Selected Titles from Seal Press

FOR MORE THAN THIRTY YEARS, SEAL PRESS HAS PUBLISHED
GROUNDBREAKING BOOKS. BY WOMEN. FOR WOMEN.

VISIT OUR WEBSITE AT: **WWW.SEALPRESS.COM**

Women Who Run by Shanti Sosienski. $15.95, 1-58005-183-9. An inspirational and informative book profiling twenty very different women and what drives them to run.

Women in Overdrive: Find Balance and Overcome Burn Out at Any Age by Nora Isaacs. $14.95, 1-58005-161-8. For women who take on more than they can handle, this book highlights how women of different age sets are affected by overdrive and what they can do to avoid burnout.

Stalking the Wild Dik Dik: One Woman's Solo Misadventures Across Africa by Marie Javins. $15.95, 1-58005-164-2. A funny and compassionate account of the sort of lively and heedless undertaking that could only happen in Africa.

Body Outlaws: Rewriting the Rules of Beauty and Body Image edited by Ophira Edut, foreword by Rebecca Walker. $15.95, 1-58005-075. Filled with honesty and humor, this groundbreaking anthology offers stories by women who have chosen to ignore, subvert, or redefine the dominate beauty standard in order to feel at home in their bodies.

Solo: On Her Own Adventure edited by Susan Fox Rogers. $15.95, 1-58005-137-5. An inspiring collection of travel narratives that reveal the complexities of women journeying alone.

Woman's Best Friend: Women Writers on the Dogs in Their Lives edited by Megan McMorris. $14.95, 1-58005-163-4. An offbeat and poignant collection about those four-legged friends girls can't do without.